S15672
618.92 Gravelle, Karen
GRA

Teenagers face to face with cancer

$11.29

DATE			

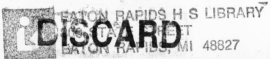

Teenagers

FACE TO FACE

WITH CANCER

Teenagers FACE TO FACE WITH CANCER

BY KAREN GRAVELLE
AND BERTRAM A. JOHN

JULIAN MESSNER ⓌⓌ NEW YORK
A Division of Simon & Schuster, Inc.

Library of Congress Cataloging-in-Publication Data

Gravelle, Karen.
Teenagers face to face with cancer.

Includes index.
Summary: Sixteen young people, fifteen of them cancer patients, describe their experiences with the disease and how they deal with family, friends, and school while coping with their illness. 1. Tumors in children—Psychological aspects—Juvenile literature.   2. Youth—Diseases—Psychological aspects—Juvenile literature.   [1. Cancer—Patients. 2. Youth—Diseases—Psychological aspects]   I. John, Bertram A   II. Title.
RC281.C4G73   1986   618.92′99′400922   86-8608
ISBN 0-671-54549-3

618.92
GRA
88/89
SHC 88
11.29

CONTENTS

CONTENTS

INTRODUCTION

Although we are listed as the authors, in a very real sense this book was written by sixteen young people, all of whom have had to cope with cancer as adolescents. Fifteen either have cancer or have recently recovered from the disease. One is the best friend of a teenage patient who died.

As a group, these adolescents come from varied backgrounds and perspectives. Of the sixteen, ten are white and six are black. They live in small towns, suburban areas, and large cities in three different states. Some of their families are well off economically, others are not. In spite of their differences, however, they all have one very important thing in common—a willingness to share their experiences openly so that the rest of us might better understand the problems of teenagers with cancer.

A few in the group wanted to use their real names in the book, but as the majority felt more comfortable remaining anonymous, we have assigned fictitious names to them all. Thus, much as we would like to, we can't acknowledge by name the adolescents who participated in writing this book. We can say, however, "You know who you are and, to you all, many thanks!"

In addition, we wish to thank several physicians and social workers who were instrumental in putting us in touch with the adolescents whose experiences are presented here and in providing us with information about the medical and psychosocial aspects of cancer. Because naming them might in turn reveal the identities of their patients, we must again say, "You know who you are, and thanks."

There is one person involved in writing the book that we can acknowledge by name, however. For her hard work, and even more, for her insight and perceptiveness, we would like to thank Caren Rabbino.

KAREN GRAVELLE
BERTRAM A. JOHN

PART ONE

THE FIRST ENCOUNTER: "I HAVE CANCER!"

In many ways, the tasks of adolescence, as a developmental stage in life, and the tasks involved in conquering cancer are on a direct collision course. Adolescence itself is problematic enough. It's a time of dramatic changes, but changes that frequently seem out of the young person's control. Everything changes—teenagers' relationships with friends, their feelings about their parents, and, most especially, their own bodies. Much of adolescence involves the struggle to understand these changes, gain some control over them, and incorporate the results into a reasonable self-image and plans for the future.

A diagnosis of cancer throws this whole process into disarray. Relationships change again and usually in a direction opposite to the one in which the adolescent had been moving. Friendships with peers are disrupted and sometimes broken, and the patient is pushed back into a position of dependence on adults for survival. Somehow, teenagers with cancer must learn to juggle the demands of adolescence with the often contradictory demands of their medical situation. How they accomplish this is the subject of this book.

But the patient isn't the only adolescent affected by the diagnosis. Friends can be hit especially hard when they hear that someone close to them has been struck by a life-threatening disease. Perhaps you are one of those friends. If so, you might identify with Carol in the following situation.

Thirteen-year-old Becky had seemed fine. There was no indication that she was sick in any way. She had developed red spots on her skin that she showed Carol, her best friend, but they didn't hurt. Then, one weekend in May, when Carol was away, Becky's brother threw a paper candy wrapper at her, making a big bruise on her mouth. Becky's parents became alarmed and called the doctor. He told them to bring her to the hospital immediately.

When Carol returned home after the weekend, Becky's older sister told her that Becky was in the hospital having blood tests. Carol was initially worried, but Becky's sister assured her it wasn't anything serious. Two days later, Carol was told that Becky had leukemia.

Carol was devastated! "People die from leukemia!" she thought. "Is Becky going to die?" As the weeks went by and Becky struggled through treatment, Carol had a lot of other questions. "How should I act around Becky?" "What can I do to help?" And, always, "Is Becky going to die?"

This book answers some of the questions that Carol had to figure out on her own. It should help you know what to expect when a friend gets cancer, how to help, and, above all, that it's all right to ask questions.

1
THE INITIAL SHOCK

*"I threw up. That's what I did. I didn't ask the
old question, 'Why me?' I just threw up."*
WINSTON

*"I was in the bathroom [of the hospital]. Dad
was holding me up. I just started crying."*
ANTHONY

It's always a shock.

Laura had been sick, in pain, and exhausted for over
a month. No one seemed to be able to figure out why
she felt so ill. Because all her joints were swollen, doctors took a blood test to check for juvenile arthritis.
They said they'd call back in a couple of days with the
results. When the phone rang only two hours later,
however, and the hospital asked Laura's parents to
bring her back the next day, everyone had an ominous
feeling that something was very wrong.

Strangely, Laura had actually wondered if she had
leukemia. Not that she thought it fit her symptoms par-

ticularly—it was just something she'd heard of. "The whole time the doctors never mentioned what they thought I had, but I was getting an X-ray taken of my leg, and I just said to my mom, 'Do they think I have leukemia?' The doctors never mentioned it 'cause they don't say anything until they're sure. I don't know where that came from." But Laura suspected her problem might be serious, and the one thing she knew about leukemia was that it was very serious. "I had watched *Something for Joey*, so I knew that people die from it and stuff." But at fifteen, that was the extent of her knowledge about the disease.

When she returned to the hospital, doctors took some of Laura's bone marrow for tests. Then they sent her and her parents to get something to eat, saying the results would be available afterward. "When we got back, they only called my mom and dad into the room, so I figured . . ." Laura sat in the waiting room for the next forty-five minutes, trying to concentrate on a magazine.

"Finally, they called me in and my mom said, 'Laura, you have leukemia.' I started crying, and my mom and dad started crying. Everyone was crying. I just asked, 'Does that mean I'm going to die?' 'cause that's what everyone thinks—that cancer means you're going to die. My mom said that they didn't know yet, that they'd have to do more tests. At that point, I just wanted to go home and say good-bye to my house and my dog and my friends for one last time. You know, go to church one last time. I thought this was it."

Winston had an inkling that he might have cancer

from something the doctor had said. Because he was having bed sweats, he had gone to his local hospital to be examined. The hematologist there wanted to do a bone marrow test to see why his white blood cell counts were going up. "They said it could be a lot of things. Then they said it could be leukemia, and they were mentioning some other things, like TB, and some other things I don't remember. I kind of knew it was leukemia, because they wouldn't have said that. I figured that's it."

When the test results did show that he had leukemia, Winston wasn't terribly upset at first. It took a while for the information to sink in. Then it hit him like a bomb! "It didn't bother me at first . . . at first. When the doctor told me, I thought, 'Wow.' I was calling up all my friends and telling them. I think I started to cry a bit over the phone. Then I got over it. No, then I threw up. That's what I did, I threw up."

Most teenagers who know anything about cancer generally know only enough to make them scared. They, like their parents, usually associate the disease with almost-certain death. The whole family shares the same initial fear—that the person with this frightening illness is going to die. Gail's mother, who is a nurse, suspected that her daughter might have cancer. Gail remembers her mother's reaction vividly. "When I got the blood count, my mom looked it over. She just started shaking. That upset me!" Cheryl's mother was as frightened as Cheryl was. "She was really scared too. She was crying, I was crying. The same thoughts were going through her head that were going through mine. 'Am I going to die?' "

Sometimes, adolescents don't recognize the words euphemistically used to refer to cancer. They, therefore, don't initially realize that others suspect they may have a malignant disease. One of these words is "tumor." When Bernadette was told she had a tumor in her stomach and had to have an operation, she wasn't concerned about the tumor itself, which she thought must be like a cyst, but about the surgery. Amy knew her mother and grandmother were very upset when X-rays of her leg indicated she had a "growth." "I didn't think it was any big deal—a growth," she said. "Nobody used the word cancer. My mom said it might be a tumor, but still no one said cancer."

Interestingly, Bernadette feels her ignorance actually worked in her favor. "If someone told me I had cancer now, I'd probably be more scared. If I got it now, I might not conquer it because of the social pressure that if you have cancer, you're going to die. I didn't have preconceptions. I just learned as I went along. Now I know that there are different kinds of cancer, with different outcomes," she adds. "Some cancers mean you're going to die, that there's no treatment."

Mixed in with the shock and the fear, there can sometimes be an element of relief on hearing the diagnosis. At least it means treatment can be started. Over the past weeks, Derek's parents had become more and more desperate. His fever fluctuated so dramatically that they were maintaining a twenty-four-hour vigil. But since nobody could figure out what was wrong with him, no one was able to help him. The day the doctors told Derek and his family that he had cancer was also the day he started to get well. Even though he had a scary, serious disease, it was more important to Derek that with treatment he was beginning to feel better.

Joel also felt a certain relief when his doctors finally decided he had cancer. Physicians at the hospital had spent six weeks trying to diagnose the problem in his leg. In the meantime, Joel had been in a lot of pain. He knew they thought he might have cancer, so he was prepared emotionally for the possibility. Although his diagnosis scared him, at least it meant the doctors could do something about his pain.

When they are told they have cancer, teenage patients are also informed about the procedures that they will go through in their treatment. Physicians are honest about the fact that chemotherapy is a long and arduous process, but patients are willing to go through it to get well. For certain patients, however, the treatment for cancer sometimes seems worse than the disease itself.

In addition to hearing that they have cancer, patients with osteogenic sarcomas, or bone cancer, learn that they may have to lose a leg in order to save their lives. For Kevin, the deal didn't seem worth it. Without his leg he could forget a career in sports. What was the point of saving his life, if the thing he lived for was impossible for him? Like Kevin, Yvonne and her family were initially much more concerned with the prospect of her leg being amputated than they were with the fact that she had cancer. For these patients and their families, the news that they had cancer was accompanied by an additional, very painful blow. Adjusting to this can take time.

When Earl heard his leg had to be amputated, he wondered, "Why? Why did this happen? Why did it happen to me?" He still doesn't know, and sometimes it still makes him angry. Amy wondered too. She thought her cancer was brought on by stress. There had been considerable emotional turmoil in her home for a few years. Kevin initially blamed his cancer on his mother. "The only thing I knew about cancer was that it was connected with smoking. My mother smoked and I thought heredity was involved, so I asked if my mother's smoking caused my cancer."

Although their doctors were able to reassure Amy and Kevin that neither her home situation nor his mother's smoking caused their tumors, physicians are unable to answer the question, "Why me?" Not being able to find a reason for the disaster that has struck their lives can be particularly difficult for adolescents to cope with.

Laura asked herself, "Why me?" a lot. "First off, who thinks you're going to get sick when you're fifteen years old? I was really confused. I went through that 'Why me?' There's no reason. I didn't smoke; I didn't drink; I didn't do drugs. I was really nice to people. There was no reason for it. It just didn't seem fair that all of a sudden I was just put into this world that I didn't belong in. I was mad and there was no one person to be mad at. You couldn't be mad at your parents or any of your friends—there was no one to be mad at, so I got angry at God. I was just real mad! I *hated* God! And when I got better, my mother put flowers in the church as a thanks offering, and I said, 'What the hell did you do that for?' And my mom said, ' 'Cause he made you better.' And I said, 'Oh, God made me better? Did he make me sick too? God only does *nice* things for people?' "

It's hard for teenagers, for anyone, to understand why they get sick. Gail is beginning to accept the possibility that she may never know. "My feelings at the beginning were the usual: Shock at first, then 'Why me?' " How does she deal with that question? "I guess you don't. You leave it unanswered, or you answer it while you grow."

PART TWO

THE AFTERSHOCK: FIGHTING BACK

Treatments for cancer vary greatly, depending on what kind of cancer is involved. In adolescents, the most common types of cancer are leukemia, non-Hodgkins lymphoma, sarcomas (particularly bone tumors), and brain cancer. The teenagers who helped in the writing of this book have (or have recently recovered from) cancers in the first three of these categories. To understand what being treated for cancer is really like, it is useful to know something about these diseases and the procedures used to treat them.

Leukemia is the term for a variety of different cancers that strike the white blood cells that originate in the bone marrow. Of the four main types of leukemia, two—acute lymphocytic leukemia (ALL), and acute myelocytic leukemia (AML)—account for almost all leukemias in children and young adults. ALL and AML are different in a number of important ways.

In teenagers, ALL is about four times more common than AML, and occurs more frequently in younger patients. Of the adolescents who contributed to this book, five were ALL patients—Dawn, Susan, Gail, Cheryl, and Laura. Thirty years ago, patients with ALL only survived for about three months after diagnosis. Primarily thanks to the discovery of new drugs, ALL is now considered one of the most curable forms of cancer.

AML, which affects a different group of white blood cells, is more common amongst older adolescents, like Winston. Unfortunately, AML is harder than ALL to treat successfully. Although doctors are usually able to induce remissions, that is, to kill the leukemia cells and restore the bone marrow, all too often the disease returns. Thus, the prognosis, or the chance of survival, is not as bright for AML patients as it is for patients with ALL.

Detecting early stages of ALL or AML can be difficult because both leukemias often resemble common infectious diseases. Fever and flulike symptoms are frequently the first signs that something is wrong. Lymph nodes can become enlarged and the person may suffer from bone or joint pain. Paleness, weakness, and a tendency to bruise easily can be other symptoms.

The usual treatment of leukemia is with chemotherapy, or cancer-killing drugs, although radiation and bone marrow transplants are sometimes also used. Chemotherapy is given in three stages. The first, induction, is the most intense, since the purpose of this stage is to destroy as many cancerous cells as possible. Different drugs are used in the second, or consolidation stage, to kill any abnormal white cells that might have survived induction. Finally, patients are placed on long-term maintenance therapy to be sure that all residual cancer cells are destroyed. The entire process takes from two to three years.

15

Another form of cancer frequently seen in adolescents is non-Hodgkins lymphoma. Derek, Anthony, Laura (yes, in addition to having ALL), Joel, and Bernadette have all been treated for this type of cancer. Although there are several types of lymphoma, all involve lymphocytes, the infection-fighting cells in the lymph nodes, spleen, and thymus. Sometimes, lymphomas also affect the tonsils, stomach, and small intestine. Because the different types of lymphoma vary greatly in terms of their symptoms, how fast they spread, and the best treatment for them, it's important to diagnose these cancers accurately.

In most cases, the first sign of lymphoma is a painless swelling in the neck, armpit, or groin caused by enlarged lymph glands; however, in some cases of non-Hodgkins lymphoma the swelling may occur in the stomach. Other symptoms include fever, night sweats, fatigue, and weight loss.

Chemotherapy, sometimes combined with radiation, is the usual treatment for patients with non-Hodgkins lymphoma. With some patients, like Bernadette, tumors can be removed surgically. Most teenage patients with non-Hodgkins lymphoma have a good chance of survival.

Finally, a number of teenagers, like Earl, Amy, Yvonne, Kevin, and Beth, develop osteogenic sarcomas, or bone cancer. Because these tumors arise in rapidly growing bone tissue, they tend to occur in the leg bones of adolescents. The first sign of osteogenic sarcoma is leg pain, often occurring in the knee. Treatment usually involves amputation of the affected part of the leg. Occasionally, however, a rod or artificial joint can be implanted to replace the removed section of bone and save the leg.

Following surgery, these patients also undergo chemotherapy to kill any cells that might have spread to other parts of the body. Because of great strides in the development of chemotherapeutic drugs, the prognosis for young people with bone cancer has improved dramatically in recent years. Treatment entails much more than merely undergoing these medical procedures, however. It also means coping with unpleasant and incapacitating side effects, learning to deal with hospitals and medical staff, and, sometimes, facing the disappointment of having treatment temporarily fail.

The following chart shows which type of cancer the teenagers who helped in the writing of this book got and when they became ill.

NAME	DIAGNOSED	RECURRENCE AGE	TYPE OF CANCER
Amy	Age 15		OS
Anthony	Age 11	12, 12½, 13, 13½	NHL
Bernadette	Age 14		NHL
Beth	Age 14		OS
Cheryl	Age 13		ALL
Dawn	Age 11		ALL
Derek	Age 12		NHL
Earl	Age 11		OS
Gail	Age 15		ALL
Joel	Age 16		NHL
Kevin	Age 11	13	OS
Laura	Age 15	18, 20	ALL NHL
Susan	Age 15		ALL
Winston	Age 18		AML
Yvonne	Age 14		OS

ALL = Acute Lymphocytic Leukemia
AML = Acute Myelocytic Leukemia
NHL = Non-Hodgkins Lymphoma
OS   = Osteogenic Sarcoma

18

2
CHEMOTHERAPY AND RADIATION

"No matter how bad it gets, sooner or later it's got to stop. The treatment, the part that's real bad, finally you don't have to go for it any more. That's when you say, 'Gee, this thing was worth it!'"

ANTHONY

"You have to face it right then and there. Chemotherapy is going to make you sick, but you're going to get better. But you can't wait till tomorrow. You have to face it as soon as the doctor tells you."

BERNADETTE

One way of attacking cancer cells is by using drugs that either kill the cells or stop them from multiplying and spreading to other parts of the body. Some drugs can penetrate, and thus destroy, cancer cells but are unable to enter normal cells. Other drugs damage the cancer cells which, unlike the normal cells, lack the ability to repair themselves. The cancer cells eventually die. Treating cancer with cell-killing drugs is called chemotherapy.

One of the advantages of chemotherapy is that it is a systemic treatment. This means that the treatment can be administered to the whole body. Since cancers such as leukemia and lymphoma are not localized in one spot, they can't be removed surgically. Fortunately, thanks to chemotherapeutic drugs, these diseases can be successfully treated.

Even patients whose tumors are removed through surgery generally undergo chemotherapy as well. In these cases, the drugs are used either before surgery, to help shrink large tumors to a more operable size, or after surgery, to kill microscopic cancer cells that might have been missed during the operation or that could have spread unnoticed to other parts of the body.

Unfortunately, chemotherapeutic drugs have disadvantages. The patient can experience a host of unpleasant side effects that can be very uncomfortable and upsetting. In Kevin's words, "Chemo was hell!" The drugs can make patients extremely nauseous. "I had a lot of trouble with chemotherapy," Amy said. "I even threw up anticipating it." Said Susan, "Sometimes it seems like it's never going to end. You look outside and see all your friends and you're just too sick or too weak from chemo to be out there."

Not all patients experience the same negative effects, however. One patient may feel deathly ill, whereas another patient, taking the same dose of the same drug, has no problem at all. At first, Laura couldn't figure out why everyone complained about chemo. "I was on three drugs and I was feeling fine. I didn't feel sick at all. I was eating like a pig. I thought, 'People really have this weird perception of what chemotherapy is. It's not bad at all.' But when they put me on another medicine,

I realized that all those stories about chemotherapy were really true. I got really, really sick to my stomach."

Chemotherapy can be administered in a number of ways. Particular treatments depend on many things—the individual, the institution, the physician, and the type of cancer involved. Even so, the following schedule is an example of how some leukemia patients are treated at one hospital. For the first five weeks, patients take pills daily and come in once a week to be given medicine through an intravenous, or IV, drip. At the end of the five weeks, the schedule changes. While they continue their daily pills, patients no longer get drugs through an IV drip but once a week through spinal taps. In the last phase of treatment, the schedule consists of daily pills, monthly injections, and a spinal tap every three months.

Spinal taps are definitely not popular. Anthony summed up his experience by saying, "There was nothing worse than that." Because medicine administered orally or through the bloodstream can't pass into the brain where cancer cells may be hiding, doctors have had to find another way of giving drugs. The spinal fluid provides a direct route into the brain, circumventing the barrier between the bloodstream and the brain tissue. Not surprisingly though, patients aren't wild about having needles inserted into their spines.

As is true with many kinds of treatment, individual patients experience spinal taps differently. Some doctors seem especially skilled at giving spinals with minimal pain, whereas others have to try several times before getting it right. Some patients, like Anthony, get

21

used to the procedure in time and aren't bothered by it anymore, whereas others find spinals increasingly difficult to tolerate. Derek had to have his last spinals under general anesthesia because the procedure had become too emotionally upsetting for him to handle. Sometimes the aftereffects of spinal taps are more problematic than the spinals themselves. As a result of the procedure, Joel had very bad headaches, which made it hard for him to function at school.

To work, chemotherapeutic drugs have to be highly effective at killing cells. Frequently, patients are frightened by the strength and possible danger of their drugs and by the feeling that they are at the mercy of the drug. One of Kevin's drugs was lethal if not administered correctly. "I was scared to death of it!" he said. Gail was afraid of chemotherapy too. "The drugs make you sick, but I think a lot of it was in my head because I was frightened. I didn't know what kind of medicine was doing what." Because Amy had such bad side effects, she felt especially helpless and unable to protect herself against the power of the drugs she was given. She hated the idea that the chemotherapy flooding into her "was going to do what it wanted to and if anything strange happens, nothing can be done about it." Undergoing chemotherapy was so difficult for her that she once pulled the IV tubes out and refused her last treatment.

Although some of the drugs used to kill cancer cells cannot penetrate healthy tissue, many of the drugs strike normal cells as well. Those particularly affected are rapidly dividing cells, such as cells in the lining of the mouth, cells in the bone marrow, and hair cells. As a result, patients on chemotherapy can have mouth sores, a depressed immune system that makes them more vulnerable to other illnesses, and hair loss. All of the normal cells do eventually come back, but in the meantime, patients have to cope with a range of problems.

Because bone marrow cells form part of the immune system's defense against viruses, bacteria, and other foreign cells, if too many marrow cells are killed off in the process of destroying cancer cells, the body is unable to protect itself against other diseases. Patients whose counts (of these immune cells) are low have to be especially careful. For some patients, none of the precautions against infection seem to work, and their lives are disrupted as much by everyday diseases as by cancer. "During the summertime, I was in the hospital at least fourteen days a month," said Laura. "Four days of chemo and then about two weeks later, I'd pick up an infection and have to go in for ten days of antibiotics, so it never stopped. I *knew* to expect an infection. I planned my life around getting chemo and then getting an infection."

Laura's experience is somewhat unusual, however. In spite of the physical effects of chemotherapy, the vast majority of cancer patients manage to stay in school and pursue normal activities while undergoing treatment. For example, in one children's hospital with approximately seven hundred youngsters (including preteenagers) in treatment, only about twenty of these are in the hospital at any one time.

The side effect of chemotherapy that is most universally hated, however, is hair loss. The majority of adolescent patients, including some who have had amputations, find this the hardest part of the entire cancer experience to deal with. As Susan points out, it hits teenagers where they feel most vulnerable. "You're really concerned with what you look like. And you look *a lot* different. I had no hair and I was a lot skinnier from being sick all the time."

With some people, chemotherapy just causes the hair to thin out. With others, hair falls out from one or two sections of the scalp. Many patients, however, go completely bald. In any event, actually seeing one's hair come out in fistfulls or waking up to find the pillow covered with hair can be especially unnerving. Winston's hair fell out at the back. He knew it looked strange and thought, "Oh, wow! Everybody's going to look at me as if I'm a freak!"

When Gail's doctor told her she might lose her hair, she thought, "I'll get a wig. It won't be so bad." She felt different when it actually happened though. "Then it started to fall out. I thought, 'Oh, God!' I mean, I have thick hair, and the doctor said it would thin out. But it thinned, and it thinned, and it thinned." Laura felt so unattractive that she worried she was making the people associated with her look bad too. "It's not just feeling ugly for yourself. It's like being introduced to your boyfriend's friends and feeling ugly for him. It just engulfs your whole world."

Although wigs can lessen much of the self-consciousness about having no hair, patients are often concerned that the wig will look funny and make them conspicuous. When she first returned to school, Gail was very apprehensive. "I thought, 'Everybody's going to know. They're all going to laugh.' But they didn't. I don't think they even noticed. I told my close friends that it was a wig, and they said, 'No, really?' "

In Anthony's case, the wig was a disaster. "The hair-dresser came over and I was fitted for the wig. I refused to wear it! It looked like *crap!* I looked better off with a hat on." Anthony was so self-conscious that he never took his hat off, even at home. For a long time, he avoided leaving the house.

Almost all teenage cancer patients express feeling painfully unattractive without their hair; but for some patients, hair loss has an additional symbolic meaning. "When you lose your hair, you really feel ugly," said Laura. "But besides feeling really ugly, it's also a constant reminder. Every day when you wake up and look in the mirror, it's like, 'Oh, my God! I'm sick!' No matter how good I feel, it's still there . . . you're bald, you're *sick!* You just can't get away from it."

Depending on the type of cancer, the severity of the disease, and the physician involved, some patients are also given radiation as another means of killing cancer cells. X-rays are directed specifically to the part of the body needing treatment, over a period of two to four weeks. Although chemotherapy can be painful, patients feel nothing during the actual process of receiving radiation. As Susan describes the procedure, "They lay you on a table and depending where you're going to get it [radiation], they put magic marker on you. You just

TYPICAL TREATMENT SCHEDULES
(Assuming there is no recurrence of disease.)

TYPE OF CANCER	TOTAL TREATMENT TIME	TYPE OF TREATMENT	TIME HOSPITALIZED
ALL	Girls—2 years Boys—3 years*	Chemotherapy (out-patient) Occasionally, 2 weeks of radiation	1 week at the start of chemotherapy
NHL	6–18 months, depending on the type of disease	Chemotherapy (out-patient, but a more intensive schedule than for ALL) Radiation for 2–4 weeks during the early part of chemotherapy	2 weeks to 1 month at the cbeginning of chemotherapy

OS	1 year	Either amputation followed by chemotherapy, or 6 weeks of chemotherapy, amputation, then the remainder of chemotherapy	Amputation— less than 1 week. Twenty 3–4 day hospitalizations for chemotherapy (amounting to about 80 out of 360 days or one quarter the year of treatment)

* Oncologists have found that girls tend to do better when treated over a two-year period, while boys do better on a three-year schedule.

lie on the table and keep your eyes closed. It only takes about five minutes."

Susan and Dawn both kept their hair throughout chemotherapy, but lost it when they had radiation. *Everyone* loses their hair if their head receives radiation. Frequently, patients who have had head radiation also experience heavy drowsiness, and sleep from twelve to fourteen hours a day for a period of two weeks to a month following treatment.

Considering the physical discomfort and emotional trauma associated with treatment, you would expect patients to be elated when the whole process is finally over. Joel's friends expected him to celebrate when his chemotherapy ended, and they were surprised and confused when Joel was most *un*excited about his new freedom. In fact, Joel was terrified. "I figured, 'Now that I'm off chemo, what's to keep the cancer from coming back? It beat me once, why not again?' " While he was on chemotherapy, Joel felt protected not only against his type of cancer but also against any other kind. Without chemo he felt completely defenseless. When his doctor told him that this was a normal, common reaction, Joel's fears began to subside. "Now," he says, "I'm in a good mood and relieved that chemo is over."

The chart on pages 26 and 27 shows typical treatment schedules for the three most common cancers that occur in adolescents.

3
AMPUTATION

"My parents were really concerned that I wasn't wearing my prosthesis, but my social worker— we're really close—told them not to pressure me."

KEVIN

"The whole world sees me with one leg. I see myself with two legs—'two legs' meaning 'fine.' I see myself as 'fine'—the whole world sees me as 'not fine.'"

BETH

Earl had complained of pain in his knee, so his mother took him to the doctor who diagnosed the problem as torn ligaments. When his leg didn't improve, Earl's mother brought him back and urged the doctor to take an X-ray. The results indicated that Earl might have osteogenic sarcoma, or bone cancer. These tumors are most frequently treated by surgical removal of the affected part of the leg. For a twelve-year-old boy who didn't know what "tumor," or even "cancer," really meant, hearing that he might lose his leg was a terrible shock.

"I started crying when my mother told me," he said. "I was scared—scared it would hurt a lot." Unfortunately, Earl's fears were realistic. Even after the operation, his amputation has continued to be painful. Earl has had considerable trouble with phantom pain, which is a common problem experienced by people who have lost a limb. The person feels pain, not from the site of the amputation itself but from the missing, or phantom, part of the body. This occurs because nerves in the brain responsible for our sense of pain continue to send out signals. Not only is this physically uncomfortable but psychologically difficult to handle as well.

Fortunately, phantom pain severe enough to require medication usually lasts only about a week. Although patients often feel sensations from the missing limb for the rest of their lives, these feelings are rarely painful. Earl's phantom pain has persisted longer than is usual. He tries to ignore it as much as possible and to get on with his life. Eventually, the phantom pain will go away.

Osteogenic sarcomas arise in rapidly growing bone tissue and therefore occur most frequently in the leg bones of adolescents. Because bone tumors are generally resistant to radiation and chemotherapy, they are usually treated surgically. Sometimes, only a small portion of bone needs to be removed and a metal rod or artificial knee joint can be implanted, thus allowing the patient to keep the leg. Most often, however, the leg must be amputated above the site of the tumor. For some patients, this is below the knee, for others, above the knee, and for some, at the hip. After the amputation site has healed, the patient is fitted with an artificial leg, or prosthesis.

Earl's prosthesis has caused some problems. Much to his mother's distress, he prefers not to wear it. "I know I have to get used to it," he says, "but it slows me down." Earl can do almost everything he did before the amputation—including riding his bike and swimming—without his prosthesis. The only time he feels he needs it is when he plays sports. His mother, on the other hand, is very anxious for him to wear the prosthesis and worries that if he doesn't get used to it soon, he may never wear it.

Kevin was initially destroyed by the loss of his leg. "The question wasn't 'Am I going to die?' but 'Why *didn't* I die? I'd *rather* die!' " Having an amputation hit him especially hard because he had been an excellent athlete and had hoped to make his career as a professional. With that possibility gone, his whole life seemed ruined. Time and the support of his parents have helped Kevin to realize that he can still have a good life, even one that includes a career in sports, as a sports journalist. In general, he now seems confident about both himself and his future.

In spite of parental pressure, Kevin also resists wearing his prosthesis. In his case, however, the problem is not just one of getting used to it. Kevin's leg was removed at the hip and his prosthesis, which weighs around twenty pounds, requires a chest harness. Besides finding it heavy and cumbersome, Kevin thinks it's ugly. "It exhausted me and bummed me out to wear it," he says. "I can move much better without it, so I never use it."

Amy can't imagine someone choosing not to wear a prosthesis. She wouldn't consider going out without hers. Not only does she feel uncomfortable without it, but she thinks not wearing her prosthesis makes people around her uncomfortable.

Initially, Amy had hoped to avoid needing a prosthesis. When she was given the option of a knee replacement, she jumped at the chance. "No way did I want an amputation!" she says. After months of complications involving infections, hospitalizations, and excruciating pain, Amy decided the knee replacement wasn't going to work. Although she was told there was a slim chance her leg could still be saved, Amy didn't think it was worth further agony and she asked her doctor to amputate. "That was the turning point. Immediately after the operation, I started to improve. I felt a lot better!"

Even though Amy preferred an amputation to struggling along with a painful, nonoperative artificial knee, it doesn't mean that she is completely happy with her prosthesis. At times, she feels self-conscious about having an artificial leg, particularly on dates. Generally, though, she thinks the problem is more in her own head than in the eyes of others.

Yvonne and her family were even more upset hearing that an amputation was necessary than they were discovering that she had cancer. Nevertheless, Yvonne seems relatively satisfied with the way things have turned out. "At first I didn't like it," she says, referring to her prosthesis. "It was heavy and it felt funny. But then it started to feel like a part of me." Yvonne really likes herself and, as her prosthesis has become integrated into her concept of that self, she's developed a genuine fondness for it as well.

Some patients, like Yvonne, seem to cope rather easily once they have made the initial adjustment to having lost a part of their body. Others have some difficulty resolving the image they have of themselves with the culturally defined image of amputees. This problem can intensify as adolescents get older and increase their contact with the larger world, where they are more directly confronted with stereotypes.

Beth's leg was amputated at fourteen and she made what she considered a good adjustment. She refused to see herself as an amputee. "I don't consider myself to be handicapped or disabled—or any of those social stereotypes. So much so that I don't identify myself with those people, with other amputees. This has led to a lot of denial on my part."

While this strategy permitted her to maintain an image of herself that was consistent with her inner reality, it led her to completely deny her outer, social reality; that is, that she is part of a culturally defined group to which negative perceptions are often attached. Beth knows exactly what these negative stereotypes are because she finds herself attaching them to other amputees.

Beth doesn't use her prosthesis, because she feels insecure and liable to fall when wearing it. Thus, it is evident even to very casual observers who see her walking on crutches that she has lost her leg. Now that she has moved to a large city, the overt stares of people on the street are making her face the fact that, however she may view herself, people in general see her as an amputee.

Beth is not the only osteogenic sarcoma patient who is ill at ease with others who have lost a leg. Amy is also very uncomfortable around amputees who don't wear a prosthesis. She thinks that she should avoid looking at them, as if viewing their condition is somehow impolite. Amy finds her own response very strange and doesn't quite know what to make of it. Like Beth, she is struggling to resolve her personal knowledge of what it's like to be an amputee together with her cultural perceptions of physically handicapped people.

Cancer has a different impact on the lives of teenagers who have amputations than on cancer patients whose disease can be treated by other means. First, it irrevocably and visibly alters their bodies at a time in life when concerns about physical appearance are most prominent. Second, it places them in a potentially stigmatizing group, "the handicapped." Third, the problems of amputations are not static but change as the adolescent matures and encounters new situations. In a sense, cancer—or more precisely, its residual effect—is never really over for these youngsters.

Now aged thirteen, Earl is worried about pain and limitations on his ability to get around. He is not yet concerned with the effect his amputation and/or prosthesis may have on his relationships with the girls he'll be dating in a few years or on his employment prospects ten years from now. The vast majority of these patients handle the problems associated with their amputations with real resourcefulness and resilience. It isn't always easy, though.

4

DEALING WITH DOCTORS

"I wanted to know what was happening, so I asked my mother. At first, I was scared to ask the doctors."

CHERYL

"I just wanted to be told everything. I didn't want to be lied to or anything."

ANTHONY

Hospitals can be very intimidating places, for parents as well as adolescents. Doctors and nurses frequently seem, if not all knowing, at least all powerful. Patients with cancer are asked to submit to mysterious, painful, and sometimes potentially dangerous procedures without being able to judge for themselves whether the person performing the procedure is competent to do it, or even whether the procedure itself is appropriate. Like other patients with serious diseases, in order to be treated, people who have cancer must give considerable control over their lives to total strangers. For adolescents, this means returning to a position of extreme dependence upon adults at the very time when, in the natural course of things, they should be in the process of establishing their independence. This sense of sudden powerlessness can be further heightened by watching their parents, previously perceived as the adults in charge, handing over control themselves and becoming dependent upon medical personnel.

Cheryl's initial experience with this confusing and remote world was not uncommon. "Doctors would come in [to the hospital room] to look at me. They were all in a group. They came and felt my neck and wrote something down. And then they left . . . I used to be real scared."

Having crowds periodically examine her and then depart made her feel like an oddity. "They made me feel like I was different . . . I got tired of them coming in and feeling my neck. They looked at me like I was strange and that's how I felt." At thirteen, Cheryl had never been in a hospital before and was too frightened to ask the doctors what was going on.

Occasionally, the patient's introduction to the hospital world can be thoroughly terrifying. "I found myself in an ambulance and then being pulled into the cold," said Anthony. "Getting to the hospital and they said, 'We don't have any beds.' Back into the ambulance, being rushed all over the place. I was scared to death because I didn't know what was going on. I thought, 'This can't be me!' I was by myself in the ambulance with mom and dad following behind."

Sometimes the initial experience is not one of fear

but of frustration. Cancer in young people can be difficult to diagnose and family doctors, who may have only
seen a few cases of cancer over the years, may not immediately recognize the disease. Kevin, Amy, and Earl
all had similar experiences when they first went to their
local doctor complaining of leg pain. The doctor didn't
think there was a serious problem. Amy's and Kevin's
physicians even suggested that they were just trying to
get attention. When, at the insistence of Earl's mother,
his doctor finally took an X-ray, it was discovered that
he had osteogenic sarcoma. Amy and Kevin were finally
diagnosed as having bone cancer too.

When Laura fell on the stairs and hurt her knee, the
pain she complained of seemed so disproportionate to
her injury that doctors thought she was faking. A
month later, when she had a rash, swollen joints, and a
high fever, they continued to question whether she
really felt as bad as she said. By this time she was too
sick to care what they thought.

Fortunately, the picture seems to improve dramatically once patients are diagnosed. Many large metropolitan areas have special facilities for treating children
and adolescents with cancer. An oncology team con-
sisting of physicians, nurses, and social workers not
only provides medical care but also helps patients and
their families deal with other problems related to
cancer. Although initially frightened of doctors at the
hospital, Cheryl warmed up to the oncology staff. All
members of the team were familiar with her case and
available to answer her questions. Kevin developed a
close relationship with his social worker, who helped

his family understand why he didn't want to wear his prosthesis.

If any one aspect can be said to be responsible for the very positive feelings teenage patients have for oncology team members, it's that the medical staff tell the truth. Over and over again, patients emphasize how important they feel this has been for them. "They were really open," said Laura. "I never got a pill without them saying to me, 'Laura, this does this and it will upset your stomach and your hair's going to fall out, but you have to have it.' They never did anything without telling me first. I'll always appreciate that. It's better than being lied to or not being told anything and just wondering."

Anthony wanted to know *everything* about his treatment and about his chances of surviving. He appreciated the way his doctors responded. "Everybody was real good. My doctor seemed to tell me as much as he could. If not, he'd come down after looking stuff up. They were always straight on the line."

For teenagers, the facts are not as scary as not knowing what to expect. "It's much more frightening when you aren't given information, when doctors and parents keep things from you," said Bernadette. She had great faith in her doctor because he explained things to her in detail. "He explained everything! Anyone who's had him will tell you that. He gives you the *cold facts*. It scares you, but you understand it."

Treating their questions and concerns with respect obviously helps adolescents feel like participants in their treatment, rather than like bodies that are being endlessly jabbed with needles. And, to the degree that knowledge equals power, patients who understand what's going on in their treatment and know what to expect have a sense of having some control over their lives. "I put my trust in the doctor," said Bernadette, "but I want to know what he's doing in case something doesn't go right."

In addition, many oncology teams are placing as much actual control over treatment as possible in the hands of patients. Patients decide which veins will be used for intravenous injections, etc., and are explicitly told, "It's your illness and you should have as much say over it as possible." Often this means only a choice between two unpleasant alternatives, but, as Derek points out, it helps to be able to say, "I don't want it [a particular treatment] at all, but if I have to have it, this is the way I'm going to have it."

Sometimes, unfortunately, the close rapport patients such as Bernadette and Anthony feel with their doctors is missing at other hospitals. Without the all-important ingredient of caring, even specialized oncology facilities don't really meet the needs of patients and their families. Earl's mother brought him from another state to be diagnosed. Alone in a strange city, she felt particularly isolated when she had to call the doctor from a pay phone in front of the hospital to get the results of Earl's biopsy. When told by a nurse she had never met that her son's leg would have to be amputated, the shock was tremendous. She had to explain the situation to Earl without the support of the doctor—a memory that is still very painful for her.

Winston has also had difficulty at his health care center. Being one of the major oncology hospitals in the country, the place is just too big to be capable of responding to him as an individual. "I've been switched to so many doctors. Some of them care, some of them are like, 'Next patient. Move them on out.' They ask questions that are real stupid to me. They ask if you're gay, if you take drugs. If I took drugs, I might as well kill myself. The object of this game, this leukemia, is to get better. If I ask for something to deal with the pain, I'm not going to get addicted. Why would anyone want to do that? I'm out there trying to make myself better."

Even under the best of circumstances, however, things occasionally go wrong. How do adolescent patients cope with the possibility that a doctor may have made a mistake, particularly if the mistake may have caused irreparable damage? Part of the problem in dealing with these situations is that it's very hard to determine when a mistake has actually been made.

Amy's family feels that the infection which resulted in the failure of her knee replacement and the subsequent amputation of her leg was somehow caused by her doctor's negligence. "My mom and grandmother were mad at the doctors. They felt the infection came from dirty tools or something the doctor did." Earl's mother states that if the local doctors to whom she brought Earl had taken his complaints seriously, valuable time wouldn't have been lost. "If the doctors had done what they were supposed to have done," she said, "maybe the cancer couldn't have been prevented, but it might not have been as bad as it was." Although aware

41

of their families' feelings on the matter, neither Amy nor Earl offers any comments of their own.

Somehow, during treatment, Anthony received what seems to be minimal spinal damage. In any event, he no longer has control over one foot and limps as a result. Since no one knows exactly what happened, it's impossible to fix blame or determine whether the damage might have been avoided.

Before her stomach tumor was discovered, Bernadette's family doctor prescribed iron supplements to correct what he thought was anemia. It now appears that these supplements may actually have facilitated growth of the tumor. "There's some possibility that the iron fed the tumor, but this is controversial," she says.

In all these cases, it's impossible to know whether the physician in fact made an error that might have been avoidable and, if so, whether that error might have caused damage. Patients are thus left unable to form an opinion as to whether or not their doctors somehow failed them. The least painful resolution of this dilemma is to assume that their doctors were competent and did their best and then to forget the issue and move on with life. This seems to be the way these adolescents have chosen to handle the situation.

5
RECURRENCE

"*I just couldn't believe it! I kept saying, 'Come on, spread it around a little! I have had more than my share!'*"

LAURA

"*I thought, 'Not again! God, why are you doing this to me?!'*"

KEVIN

"I was on chemotherapy for two and a half years, through most of high school. When I finally got to stop my medicine, I took all my friends out to dinner and had a nice celebration. I never thought I'd get sick again!" But the following November, right in the middle of midterms, Laura discovered she had developed a strange lump. As soon as exams were over, she went to the doctor.

"I couldn't believe it! I had a totally new type of cancer. This wasn't a recurrence of my leukemia. It was non-Hodgkins lymphoma. I was worse than angry that time! I refused treatment for three weeks. I said, 'I just went through this for two and a half years and I'm not going to go back on it again!' " However, when a friend of hers who had also refused treatment died, Laura changed her mind.

After some very scary months when none of her medications seemed to work, Laura's disease finally responded to a new experimental drug. This time when treatment ended, Laura didn't celebrate. "Then I stopped my medicine and I was really scared. I was paranoid all the time, always checking myself for lumps. Every little sign of a lump or an ache brought back all these memories of being sick, and I was really scared—all the time, every day."

Nevertheless, when her leukemia recurred ten months later, Laura was completely unprepared for the news. "I was totally floored! I was feeling *fine* and didn't have any reason to even *suspect* I was sick. Then, oh, my God! It's back again!" Now in her sophomore year in college, Laura's cancer is under control again, although she is still on medication. Her plans for the future have become rather tenuous, however. After all, she doesn't know what to expect anymore.

Having a recurrence of the disease they fought so hard to conquer is a demoralizing and frightening experience for cancer patients of any age. But for teenagers eager to make up for lost time and full of plans for the future, it is particularly difficult. No matter how well they handled the question of "Why me?" when they first got sick, having to deal with a recurrence frequently leaves adolescent patients feeling singled out for persecution. A recurrence also forces patients to truly face the possibility, often for the first time, that they may not live. Kevin had been off chemo for almost two years when a tumor was found in his lung. Like Laura, he was stunned and angry. "It also made me think, 'Sooner or later, I'm going to die.'"

Typical of many patients who have struggled through years of treatment only to find that their disease hadn't been conquered after all, Kevin wondered whether it was worth going through the whole experience again. "I think what made me go on was the two years I'd had of being well, when I learned I could still do almost anything I wanted or be what I want." So he too returned to treatment.

Perhaps because Kevin has had no further problems since he recovered from this second bout of cancer, having experienced a recurrence doesn't appear to have changed his perspective on his life and his future. It has had a dramatic effect on the way Laura views things, however. For her, cancer has taken on some of the qualities of a long-term chronic illness. It is getting increasingly difficult for her to imagine ever being rid of cancer, and the possibility that she may get sick again shapes her plans for the future.

This is particularly true in terms of her plans for a family: "I'd really love to be just a mother. Even if I can have kids, though [there is some question about the side effects of chemotherapy on her reproductive system], I don't know if I ever would. Because what if I die? I would never want to put my kids through that."

Right now, Laura's plans for the future are held in

45

abeyance. "I'm due to stop my medicine in a couple of years. I think the year after that will decide a lot about my attitude toward the future . . . If I get sick again, I wouldn't get married and I wouldn't have kids 'cause I wouldn't put the emotional stress on anyone to go through that."

In the meantime, she deals with problems associated with any long-term on-and-off illness. For Laura, one of the most upsetting aspects of being chronically sick has been the effect it has had on her relationships with boyfriends. Coping with a serious disease year in and year out can be emotionally wearing on family and friends as well as on the person who is sick. Unlike the patient, however, who can't walk away from the disease (and family, who don't), friends can, and sometimes do, decide that enough is enough. "I just broke up with a guy I'd been going out with for three and a half years. His reason was that he was just tired of going through my being sick."

Anthony has also suffered multiple recurrences, but their effect on him has been different. Not that he wasn't angry and hurt. "When I was told I had a marrow recurrence, I just hollered at the doctor." But Anthony doesn't seem to see his recurrences as an indication that he might not make it. It's beginning to look as if he might be right. "The doctors really don't know how to explain his success right now," his mother says. "He's so much healthier than other patients whose counts are much better. He's defied the medical books."

Recurrences affect not only the patients who experience them but other patients as well. Watching cancer recur in a friend, with whom a teenage patient has identified, can have a powerful impact. Not only does the adolescent patient fear losing the friend, but the friend's recurrence is sometimes felt to be an omen of the patient's own future health. Joel identified strongly with another boy at his clinic. Although this boy had a different type of cancer, Joel felt they were very much alike. "We started treatment at the same time, we had the same schedule, we went through everything together. He was another nice Jewish boy like me." When the other boy had a recurrence, Joel thought that somehow this meant that he was also going to get sick again.

The majority of adolescent cancer patients do not experience a recurrence of their disease. Nevertheless, the knowledge that it's possible makes most patients very concerned that it could happen to them. Checkups are understandably a time of anxiety, as they bring the whole issue out in the open again.

Amy has been off chemotherapy for two years now. Most of the time, she feels pretty confident about her health, but occasionally, especially before her clinic appointments, she worries. "In fact, I'm overdue [for a checkup] now, but I've been putting it off because it makes me nervous." Amy had a dream recently in which she had cancer in her other leg. In her dream, she refused to have it amputated. When she woke up, she wondered what she'd do if that really happened.

PART THREE

RELATIONSHIPS WITH OTHERS

Perhaps the most important area of concern for adolescents is their relationships with others. In an effort to grow up and become independent from their parents, they invest their emotional energy in relationships with people their own age, and these relationships assume great importance. Having cancer can put an incredible stress on these vital friendships, sometimes straining them to breaking point. Relationships with adults change as well. The usual rebellion against adult authority figures, typical of this period of life, is a luxury teenagers with cancer cannot afford if they want to survive. Also, assaults on their bodies, and subsequently their body images, can hamper their efforts at establishing romantic relationships with others of the opposite sex. The fact that most adolescent patients manage to bounce back, overcoming these obstacles, is truly a tribute to their faith and ingenuity.

6
PARENTS

"I didn't want to be a burden on my mom. I didn't want her to think she had to take care of me. I was going to conquer it myself. If I couldn't do it myself, I wasn't going to do it at all."

BERNADETTE

"My mom's always been, and still is, very scared that I'm going to die, and it makes her cling to me a lot . . . I wish she could break away a little more."

LAURA

At fourteen and fifteen, Bernadette and Laura were enjoying their new sense of freedom and their ability to take increasing control over their own lives. Then, WHAM! All of a sudden, nothing seemed to be under their control. With the diagnosis of cancer, their independence disappeared overnight and their relationships with adults went into reverse. Instead of two teenagers beginning to break away from their parents and to challenge adult authority figures, they had become two girls dependent on medical personnel for their lives and desperately needing their parents for emotional support.

Although most adolescents experience some ambivalence about leaving childhood to become adults, having cancer throws this struggle into sharp relief. For the reality is that a cancer patient is *not* independent, and rebellion against the dictates of adults can be suicidal. Bernadette and Laura, like most teenagers with cancer, managed to handle their conflicting needs to be independent and to be taken care of, while fighting to get well at the same time.

Bernadette responded to imposed dependence by grabbing back as much control over her life as she could, and, for Bernadette, knowledge meant power. She questioned the medical staff in detail about every procedure, every medication, every potential side effect, and demanded that the answers be in technical terms, not "baby words." Unlike her mother, who "wasn't the type to research things," Bernadette aggressively hunted down every fact pertaining to her illness and became the person that other family members (her mother and adult brother and sister) came to for information.

In spite of her fierce drive to be independent, however, and her success at getting everyone involved to treat her like an adult, there were times when Bernadette wanted a parent to lean on. The same young woman who said that she didn't want her mother to take care of her needed very much to be taken care of occasionally, something her mother fortunately sensed. "My mom could have dropped me off [at the hospital] for chemo and come back later to get me, but she didn't. She stayed the whole time, even when I fell asleep. She was there—just because I needed her, she was there."

Finding the balance between dependence and independence has been harder for Laura and her family, partly because of the severity of her illness. Not only was Laura sicker than Bernadette, but she was sick for a much longer period of time. Repeated stays in the hospital, over the years, disrupted relationships with her friends and made her rely more and more on her family for emotional support. Laura and her mother became very close when she was hospitalized. "My heart swells up whenever I think about how much love my mom has for me . . . Her life stopped when I got sick. She stayed with me in the hospital, put her bed right next to me. She used to get up at five in the morning to go to work. She would go home and then come right to the hospital. She was there *every single night* for four to five months."

It's clear that Laura cherishes her mother for having provided support when she so badly needed it, but now that she's out of the hospital and back at school, Laura finds her mother's concentrated attention stifling. "I don't think I'm too happy that it [her illness] encompasses my mom's life now. Sometimes, she'll get on the phone and she doesn't even want to talk—she just wants to know that I'm on the other end." Feeling trapped between her love for her mother and her desire to establish a separate life of her own, Laura was able to convince her family that they needed to join her in seeing a family counselor.

Sometimes, the problem a young cancer patient

faces in dealing with parents is not too much attention but too little. Amy's parents are divorced and she lives with her mother and step-father. When her father was informed that Amy might have cancer, he seemed unconcerned. "My father and that side of the family kept saying, 'Don't worry, it's nothing. Everything will be fine.'" When things turned out not to be fine and Amy's leg was amputated, her father's response was, "She can handle it. She's strong." Amy is strong and has handled it, but it would have been much easier for her if she thought her father had cared.

Obviously, when divorced parents live hundreds of miles apart, it is easier for the parent with whom the child lives to provide day-to-day support during a long illness. Unfortunately, even when both parents still reside in the same community, other obstacles may prevent the noncustodial parent from "being there emotionally" during rough treatment periods. Heavy involvement with a very sick child over long periods of time inevitably means having to deal in an emotionally charged context with an ex-spouse, something both parents may be anxious to avoid.

In other situations, a parent who has built a new life may wish to maintain some emotional distance from the old one. Although Laura, like Amy, received tremendous support from her mother, she needed her father as well. What she experienced as his lack of interest has permanently altered her feelings for him. "I was in the hospital those five months and he'd come to visit me once a week 'cause he had to visit his girlfriend . . . So during those years [when she had cancer], he destroyed whatever relationship we had."

Even in intact families, some parents have great difficulty giving emotional support to a child with cancer. Overwhelmed by feelings of guilt, helplessness, and anger, these parents may attempt to cope with their own emotional pain by denying the reality of their children's condition. Unfortunately, maintaining this denial requires a parent to keep an emotional (and sometimes physical) distance from the sick child.

Teenagers with cancer need all the support they can get, but not all cancer patients want the same kind of support. "When I got cancer," said Kevin, "I became a little bastard. I blamed my parents, I fought the nurses, I was all caught up in the question of 'Why me?' " His parents understood his anger and hung in there with him. "My family really pulled me through. My parents were always strong in front of me. They helped me see I could still do something with my life even if I wasn't going to be an athlete."

It can be hard for parents to find the right balance between encouraging an adolescent cancer patient's independence and providing enough emotional support, especially when the patient may not be too sure what he or she wants. Most families manage to find a happy medium that fits the current situation. "When I go into the hospital," says Laura, "I revert to being a kid again. My mom does all these things for me. Then I go home and my mom and I talk about guys and stuff."

7

BROTHERS
AND SISTERS

*"We're always arguing. So his way to get back
at me is to say, 'I can't wait for that thing
[cancer] to get you! Then I'll have all your
clothes and everything.'"*

WINSTON

*"My parents were on vacation when the doctors
found another tumor. They were going to be
back in a week, so I didn't want to call them
and spoil everything. Me and Marie—that's
my sister—were sitting on my bed and we just
started crying. She held me and said everything
would turn out OK."*

ANTHONY

How other children in a family respond to a brother
or sister with cancer depends on a number of factors.
Not the least of these is the type of relationship the
children had before the disease struck. "I'm my father's
favorite of all his kids," said Winston. "He has six
kids, but I'm his favorite, according to him." When his
younger brother tells him, in essence, that he wishes
Winston would die, Winston shrugs it off, saying,
"That's his way." The two brothers have never been
close, and their father's increased involvement with

Winston, as a result of his having cancer, has only sharpened the younger boy's long-standing jealousy.

In contrast, Anthony and his older sister have always been close. Talented, popular, and outgoing, she had frequently included him in the glamorous activities of 'the big kids.' A protective, affectionate older sister before Anthony got sick, she remains so now, and Anthony reciprocates with near total adoration.

Most adolescents and their siblings are neither as distant as Winston and his brother nor as close as Anthony and his sister. Instead, they feel a mixture of love, annoyance, rivalry, and friendship for each other. When a teenager develops cancer, both new strains and new strengths can surface in his or her relationship with brothers and sisters.

In spite of being only a year apart in age, Laura and her sister, Joanne, were not especially close. The fact that their father made no bones about his preference for Laura helped to place a barrier between the two girls. But when he moved out of the home and Laura developed leukemia, the barrier disappeared. "Joanne's different because she understands. It's almost as if she goes through it [having cancer] too. She's there all the time and she just *knows* everything . . . She's my best friend."

In other instances, a sibling may be struggling with his or her own separate problems. Having to deal with someone else's illness may complicate the sibling's ability to handle these other problems. Dawn's family, for example, has experienced more than its share of health problems. Her grandmother has diabetes and its complications have caused her to lose both legs. Dawn's sister, Brenda, also has diabetes and a younger brother is blind in one eye. In the middle of all this, Dawn was diagnosed as having leukemia. The family is a warm and caring one and Dawn is close to her many brothers and sisters. Brenda's friends, however, claim that the girls' mother treats Dawn better than she does Brenda. From Dawn's perspective, this isn't true. "My momma treats all her kids the same. She has no pets. We're all her kids. Nobody gets more."

Having fought hard for her own life, Dawn is confused and angry when her sister refuses to take her insulin, eats excess sugar, and goes into a coma. Is Brenda making a purposeful play for more parental attention? Is she jealous of the family's focus on Dawn? Possibly. But at sixteen, Brenda is also an adolescent trying to achieve her own independence while coping with the restrictions imposed by a chronic and limiting disease. In many respects, her struggle is similar to, but not necessarily caused by, Dawn's situation.

It's not unusual for the brothers and sisters of cancer patients to feel neglected by their parents and jealous of the concentrated attention received by the sick child. Realistically, caring for a child with cancer can take up the lion's share of parents' time and concern, leaving other children in the family with less support at the very time when they are experiencing more stress. In addition, since their concerns often seem trivial compared to the patient's problems, siblings frequently feel guilty about wanting more of their parents' attention.

This may be less of a problem for the family of an adolescent cancer patient than for the family of a younger patient, however. If, like Anthony, Derek, Bernadette, and Laura, the adolescent is the youngest child in the family, older brothers and sisters have reached the point where they are at least partially self-sufficient and are less likely to feel deprived of parental attention.

Moreover, teenage cancer patients are able to take more responsibility for their own treatment. This enables their parents to spend more time and energy on the other children in the family. At fifteen, Cheryl was determined to go by herself to her clinic appointments. "She insisted on going alone, so I let her," said her mother with a smile. Laura has also been able to assume more responsibility for herself and her treatment with each bout of cancer. "When I was fifteen, my parents decided what medicine I was going on, when I could come home from the hospital, all those things. Then when I was eighteen, I said I didn't want treatment anymore [she later changed her mind] and my parents couldn't make me because I was old enough to make my own decision. My mother used to give me my pills. Now when I go home, I take my antibiotics and, if not—well, then I don't."

Sometimes, being part of a very large family helps both the patient and his or her siblings deal with the disruption cancer has caused in their lives. Kevin has five brothers and two sisters. "There are eight kids in my family, so there was *always* someone there when I needed them, always someone to visit me in the hospital." Kevin and his brothers and sisters also had plenty of prior experience in sharing their parents' attention and in turning to each other for support.

Occasionally, having a brother or sister with cancer heightens siblings' fears of developing the disease themselves. Although they know that cancer is not contagious, these children are aware that the disease can "run in families." Particularly in the case of older siblings with some understanding of heredity, a brother or sister with cancer may be perceived as evidence that relatives, including themselves, are vulnerable. At twelve, Earl developed cancer. His sixteen-year-old sister admits, "Yeah, I wonder if that means I'll get it too, or maybe my kids. After all, my grandma had it and now Earl." This seems to be an especially difficult question for siblings to discuss, possibly because they feel that, even if their fears are justified, there is nothing that can be done about it.

8

FRIENDS

*"In the beginning, I was afraid of how my
friends would react. I expected them to treat
me different, like I was special because of the
leukemia, instead of being just me. I didn't
want that!"*

GAIL

*"My friend Tom is the most important person
to me besides my parents. Some of my other
friends didn't hang out with me that much
anymore because I couldn't play sports or do a
lot of stuff like I used to, but Tom was there
through everything."*

KEVIN

For teenage cancer patients, as well as healthy adolescents, relationships with friends are of critical importance. In addition to providing companionship and
recreation, these relationships are a vital source of emotional support as young people begin to assert their
growing independence from parents. Friendships with
others their own age provide mirrors that let adolescents see what their newly formed, and still shaky, self-
images look like to others. Disruptions in these important relationships are traumatic for any teenager, but
they are particularly painful for adolescents with
cancer.

61

At precisely the time when they are most concerned with their acceptability in the eyes of others, teenagers with cancer are faced with having a negative image—that of cancer patient—superimposed on them. Almost to a person, they respond by vigorously rejecting that image as part of their identity and by demanding that others perceive them as they see themselves—that is, as the same people they were before they got sick. Susan's comment is typical of the hope that friends will look beyond the fact that she has cancer. "You really don't change that much. Just your appearance changes. *You're* still the same person. Sometimes people don't understand that."

Typically, rumors spread that exaggerate their condition and paint these patients as being at death's door. "It's funny how some people think," said Derek. "As soon as they hear something and it gets spread around, it changes. Somebody said, 'He had a heart transplant.' They went crazy with it." He was anxious to correct these misconceptions and tried to encourage friends to talk with him about his illness. "I wanted friends to ask me about it. Really, you're *waiting* for them to ask you. You know if you've been out of school that long they're curious. And you want them to know the truth, instead of a lie or something."

Perhaps most upsetting to these young people is the idea that friends and classmates see them as dying. Bernadette worked hard to persuade her friends that she wasn't an invalid or on her way to the grave. "Friends who knew someone or had a grandparent with cancer expected me to lie around being sick or waiting to die. I had to convince them that I was OK, that I could go places and do things and I wouldn't get hurt."

Joel tries to show friends that his illness isn't the only thing in his life by making jokes about cancer. When his hair began to fall out at a party, Joel handled the situation by laughingly pulling it out in clumps. Although many of his friends are unnerved by his jokes, he feels it's important to demonstrate "that cancer isn't so terrible, that it doesn't command my life."

Almost all teenage cancer patients want their friends to ask questions. This not only breaks the ice, but allows patients some control over the way their experience is presented and how it is perceived by others. Friends, on the other hand, often mistakenly feel that their questions will be intrusive or painful to the patient. As Susan recalls, "They were kind of reluctant to ask me about it. They figure you're having a tough time as it is, that maybe you don't want to talk about it, but that's not true." Gail's experience is similar. "A couple of my friends come up to me and talk about things like my medications. Some of them seem afraid. I guess they don't want to get me upset. But I'm glad when they're interested."

Talking about their experiences with friends also helps teenage patients deal with the tremendous stress involved in undergoing treatment, having their lives disrupted, and facing the possibility of death. "No matter how many times someone repeats it [information about cancer], the next time they repeat it, they

63

might feel like more pressure has been let off them," says Anthony. "Talking to someone else, another friend, is always good!"

Winston relies on one friend in particular for support. "I have a friend that I talk to, say, twenty-four hours a day. He's there when I need someone. He's a friend, a best friend. It's mostly that he's available to listen." And, as Susan says, "Sometimes, if you're really down, your friends can help you feel better."

Important as these relationships are, maintaining them is not always easy. The sicker the adolescent is and the longer he or she is out of school and removed from everyday activities, the greater the gap between the patient's life and that of friends. As time passes, healthy teenagers move on with their lives, increasingly forgetful of their sick friend with whom they have less and less in common. Anthony was out of school for two years. Watching his friends drift away was very upsetting for him. "I felt like a lot of people didn't care. Nobody called. So I knew who my friends were—nobody called."

Kevin had a similar experience, but while he lost some friends, he gained a new, very special one. Before getting sick, Kevin's friendships centered on sports. When, after his amputation, he could no longer engage in these activities, many of his friends quit coming around. To his surprise, however, one boy on his baseball team, not someone Kevin had been especially close to, hung in there with him "through everything." Kevin has made other friends now, but Tom is still the most important person next to his parents for him.

Sometimes, having cancer places more subtle barriers between the patient and friends. Although the term "cancer patient" has, in general, negative connotations, certain aspects of the experience can make the patient the center of some very flattering attention. As Laura said, "I used to tell people that I was sick just because everyone thinks you're so wonderful when you tell them. They say, 'My god, how can you go to school and work at a job if you have cancer?!' And you think, 'Oh, I am great, aren't I?' I used to tell people I was sick just so they could say how great I was." Gail wants her friends to ask questions about her illness because it indicates they're interested. But she also likes the way it places her in the role of expert. "I enjoy it. I feel like I'm smarter."

By desiring feedback that acknowledges their difficult struggle and reassures them that they are valued and admired, teenage cancer patients occasionally begin to cultivate a heroic image. Because she beat terrible odds and survived a fatal disease, Beth was seen by her family and friends as "a fourteen-year-old blessed angel"—an image she readily adopted. Although seeing oneself glorified in the eyes of friends may help compensate for feelings of ugliness and social isolation, these overly positive images can backfire, pushing friends further away, as Laura discovered. "But it also put me on a different plane than they were, because all of a sudden, any problem they had—the worst problem in their life—was nothing when I said, 'I have to go into the hospital this weekend.' Their hair not working out, the guy they're going out with this weekend—

they thought I just wouldn't think it was important."

On rare occasions, an adolescent patient may decide to keep the fact that he or she has cancer confidential. Because cancer generally involves long absences from school or visible indications of the nature of the disease, this is not usually an option for teenage cancer patients. Cheryl told only her best friend that she had cancer. Classmates know that she goes to the hospital once a month, but they do not know for what she is being treated. "I don't like telling my business," she says. "It should stay in the family."

Finally, friends are not just other adolescents who either support or fail to support a cancer patient, but people who themselves are affected, sometimes profoundly, by their friend's illness. Since both parties of a close friendship rely on the emotional support it provides, disruption of that relationship can be as upsetting to the healthy person as to the one who has become sick. When Becky developed leukemia, Carol was terrified. "I was afraid that she would die or that things would change between us. I wanted everything with us to stay the same!" The two girls managed to maintain their relationship unchanged while Becky was sick. Carol came to the hospital every day after school, and she and Becky hung out and talked as always. Carol desperately needed her friendship with Becky and made the long trip back and forth from the hospital as much for herself as for her sick friend. And, in doing so, she provided the mainstay of Becky's emotional support.

9

BOYFRIENDS AND GIRLFRIENDS

"I didn't want to go with anyone because I didn't want to burden them with my problems."

SUSAN

"Yeah, my amputation's made me worry more about being rejected."

KEVIN

Many adolescent cancer patients have not started dating or are not involved with anyone special when their disease is first diagnosed. For those teenagers who do have a boyfriend or girlfriend, however, getting cancer can sometimes mean the end of that relationship.

Amy and her boyfriend encountered a number of problems when she developed osteogenic sarcoma. "My parents thought we should break up. They didn't think I could handle it all. And my boyfriend and my mom didn't get along. He accused her of causing it [Amy's cancer] because she divorced my father. It got so they weren't talking."

Amy's hometown was over fifty miles away from the large metropolitan hospital where she was treated, and the geographical separation from her boyfriend helped to increase the emotional distance between them. Since her boyfriend didn't have a car, it was difficult for him to visit her. Also, because he and Amy's mother weren't speaking to each other, he couldn't get a ride with her family when they came to the hospital or call them for information about her. Although he occasionally contacted her father to find out how she was doing, as time passed he drifted further and further away.

Amy feels that there were other factors, more directly connected with her having cancer, that also helped bring an end to the relationship. "I think it was hard for him to look at me when I was in the hospital. I just looked *so different.* I was down to sixty-eight pounds, I had no hair, and I was always in such pain."

Laura experienced similar problems in her relationship with the boy she had been dating. "My boyfriend broke up with me because he said I was being too dependent. I was in the hospital for five months and I wanted him to be there all the time. He just said he couldn't deal with it all. That really hurt! I mean, at the worst point in your life, when you think you're going to die, and then you get dumped too. . . ."

Although she didn't know it at the time, Laura's boyfriend was struggling with other problems that made it harder for him to handle having a seriously ill girlfriend. "Well, I found out later that his mother also had cancer, so he was going through it at home and then with me too. But he never told me. I went out with him for eight months and he never, ever said anything."

The problems Amy and Laura faced in maintaining relationships with their boyfriends may have been more pronounced than for many cancer patients. Both girls were particularly sick. Lengthy stays in the hospital increased the time Amy was separated from her boyfriend and resulted in Laura placing increasing emotional demands on her boyfriend. In addition, their boyfriends had problems of their own that made it hard for them to reach out in the ways these girls needed.

Even in less severe cases, however, it can be difficult for any adolescent to deal with the stress and emotions that arise when a boyfriend or girlfriend gets cancer. Susan feels that some boys may not want to get too close to someone with a serious illness. "There was one guy from last year . . . We were getting to like each other and this year I think he shied off because I have leukemia. Maybe he doesn't want to get too involved with the whole thing. If he goes out with me, then he has to worry about what I'm going through. With someone else, he doesn't."

Romantic relationships between healthy teenagers frequently break up. Thus, it shouldn't be surprising when relationships subjected to additional pressures also fall apart. Unfortunately, for the cancer patient, this can just add to the sense of feeling abandoned and of losing control over the important things in life.

When they first return to school, many teenage cancer patients are somewhat shy about dating. Because of chemotherapy, they frequently have no hair, which makes them extremely self-conscious. Although most wear wigs until their hair grows back, they often still feel painfully unattractive. "At first I thought no one would like me because I didn't have any hair," Joel remembers. "When I found out that this one girl liked me, I jumped at the chance. I kind of thought it was her or nothing. But after a while, I realized I really didn't like her all that much. Later, I met someone new that I really liked. When I told her I had a wig on, she said, 'So what?' Other girls I met knew about it and it didn't make a difference to them either."

Having already lost a boyfriend because of her illness, Laura wondered whether *anyone* would like her. "I'd had that guy break up with me, so I'd had a bad experience. I thought everyone was going to be like that and I'd have to sit all by myself at lunch. But my old friends were still my friends and I dated the guy who was the center of the football team."

For most teenagers with cancer, problems about dating are only temporary. Once off treatment and feeling well, they find that their history of cancer makes little difference to their social life. As their hair and weight return to normal, so does their confidence. Dawn finished treatment when she was fourteen. In the year since then, she has met a boy that she really likes. Dawn and her boyfriend are very close emotionally and he regrets that he didn't know her when she had leukemia. He feels his support could have helped when she was going through a rough time.

Like Dawn, most ex-patients find that their lives, including their relationships with boyfriends and girlfriends, are no different from the lives of teenagers who never had cancer. If they see any changes in the way they relate to others, they almost invariably view these changes as positive. Often they feel more sensitive to other people and their problems.

Teenagers from one group, however, frequently continue to feel some degree of discomfort in relating to others, especially in terms of dating. Unlike most patients who have completed treatment, these adolescents have been left with visible and permanent alterations to their appearance. Usually, although not always, they had osteogenic sarcomas that required amputation.

Objectively, Amy admits that her amputation and prosthesis haven't seemed to seriously affect how boys view her. The fact that she has lost a leg certainly hasn't stopped them from asking her out. Even when her date has not known ahead of time, it hasn't seemed to have made a difference to him. It makes a big difference to Amy, though. "There are so many things I can't do, especially in the summer, like swimming and going to the beach and stuff. If I'm going out with a guy, lots of times I wonder if he'd rather be with someone who can do all these things. Last summer I went to the beach with a guy. Everyone was in shorts and bathing suits and I was in jeans. I just started crying 'cause I can't do what everyone else is doing." Technically, of course, Amy can go swimming, but the one time she tried, she felt so self-conscious that she's not willing to do it again. Even when dressed like everyone else, she sometimes finds herself preoccupied with her prosthesis. "When I go out with someone new, I worry about whether it will squeak or something. I think, 'What if he *touches* it?' "

In Amy's opinion, amputations are harder for girls to cope with because of the greater importance of appearance for girls. But, boys report feeling similar effects on their relationships as well. Kevin has always been shy about asking girls out, but his amputation has made him more reluctant to risk rejection. He solves this problem by waiting for girls to come to him. "I have relationships with girls, but they have to take the initiative," he says.

Although Anthony did not have an amputation, treatment for his cancer resulted in spinal cord damage that left him with no control over his right ankle and foot. Because he limps noticeably, he feels that his altered appearance affects how other people perceive him. "I wish that other kids wanted to be as popular with me as I want to be with them. I wish I looked different, that I could walk straight so I could be popular."

Unfortunately, these feelings of insecurity and unattractiveness attached to having a visible physical liability do not always lessen with time. For Beth, the problems arising from her amputation have intensified as she has become older and her relationships with boyfriends have become more physically intimate and emotionally complex. "I would say, generally, that guys my own age find that I represent a problem for them. If they reject me, they have to prove to themselves that they are not rejecting me on the basis of my having one leg, even if they are. And if they love me, they also have to prove they don't love me on the basis of my one-leggedness."

Happily, others who have undergone an amputation have been able to incorporate this change into a body image they can feel proud of, or at least comfortable with. If some people, including prospective dates, can't accept the way they are, then perhaps those individuals aren't worth having as friends. "Hey," says Yvonne, referring to her prosthesis, "it's part of *me*. If they don't like it, then they don't like me and that's just too bad."

Some adolescents with amputations make statements like this more as a challenge to others than as an expression of their real feelings. In Yvonne's case though, it seems to reflect a genuine acceptance of her body and of the way she looks. Perhaps a critical factor in Yvonne's adjustment has been the fact that her prosthesis has come to actually *feel* like part of her body and not like an alien object attached to her. Unlike Beth, who, when she dreams never sees her leg missing or her crutches, Yvonne has managed to incorporate her altered body into her internal picture of herself.

10
PROBLEMS AT SCHOOL

*"Out of the clear blue sky, the teacher picked
the topic, cancer, and looked straight at me!"*

BERNADETTE

*"She said, real loud, in front of the class, 'Is it
because of your disease that you're doing
that?' "*

WINSTON

On the whole, adolescents with cancer seem to feel
that people in their lives treat them with dignity, com-
passion, and understanding. Teachers are generally de-
scribed by teenage cancer patients as helpful adults
who manage to respond to the teenager's medical problems with flexibility, without making the patients
themselves feel unnecessarily different. The adolescent
patients involved in the writing of this book related
only two incidents in which they felt that someone had
been inexcusably insensitive or, even worse, purposely
hostile to them in connection with their having cancer.

Thus, it is surprising that both incidents involved high school teachers.

Understanding these events is difficult. They sound (at least to a detached adult) more like very clumsy slips than like vicious attacks. Yet, the adolescents involved perceived both incidents as much more than mistakes, and continue to be upset by the memories of them. For this reason, it seems worthwhile to examine them both in the hope that similar occurrences can be avoided in the future.

Bernadette had never been particularly reticent about the fact that she had cancer. She even talked about her illness in front of her biology class. She knew that many people were uninformed about the disease and, if they were genuinely interested, she was more than happy to help others learn about cancer and how it is treated.

Although no one discussed it openly, Bernadette knew her gym teacher also had cancer. The physical signs were unmistakable to someone with Bernadette's experience. Finally, a short time before she died, the teacher approached Bernadette and wanted to talk. Bernadette was glad that she could give her moral support.

When it came to another school situation, however, in which she was publicly identified as a cancer patient, Bernadette felt entirely different. "We had to pick a topic for a research paper and out of the clear blue sky, the teacher picked the topic, cancer, and *looked straight at me!* I didn't know how to handle it! All the other kids knew she was nagging at me. Later, everyone asked me why I didn't walk out of class, but I didn't want to give her the satisfaction of thinking she'd hurt me . . . I complained to the superintendent. I didn't want her to be punished—I just wanted her to know that I realized what she did." Bernadette did her paper on child abuse. "This was the only time I ever wanted to avoid talking about cancer," she said. Although the teacher could certainly be accused of being boorish, it's not clear that she actually meant to hurt Bernadette. Yet, not only Bernadette but others in the class felt this was the teacher's intent.

Although Winston's friends all know that he has leukemia, he keeps a much lower profile than Bernadette. Nevertheless, he can tolerate friends calling out, "Hey, leukemia boy," in the middle of a crowded school hall in an effort to get his attention. When a teacher drew attention to him as a cancer patient, however, he found the incident very upsetting.

"I gave the teacher a letter saying I had leukemia. The medicine was making me really drowsy in class. We were working, and I was done and waiting for more instructions. I guess I dozed off for a second. She said, real loud, in front of the class, 'Is it because of your disease that you're doing that?' Everybody looked at me like, 'What does he have?' I thought, 'Oh, wow! That was mean!' " Winston was so angry that he complained about the teacher's behavior to the school administration. For someone like Winston, who hates to make waves over anything, this was a big step.

Neither Bernadette nor Winston considered talking

directly to the teacher about her behavior and how it had affected them. Since both adolescents believe that the teacher knew the effect her actions would have, what would have been the point? In fact, as far as Bernadette was concerned, it would only have given the teacher the pleasure of knowing she had really hit the mark.

The similarities between the two incidents provide some clues as to the sort of things teachers of teenage cancer patients might avoid. First, while most adolescents are very willing to answer questions about their disease and may, like Bernadette, even be comfortable talking in front of the class about their experience with cancer, they do so because they want people to understand their situation. Assuming the role of public cancer patients is acceptable *only* when they feel that the attention this focuses on them arises from a genuine interest on the part of other people. Being singled out publicly as a cancer patient, without this sense of concern and interest, leaves teenage patients feeling stripped and humiliated. Moreover, it is perceived by adolescents in this situation as an overtly hostile act.

Second, teenagers need to feel a certain amount of control over those situations in which they are willing to be public cancer patients. For adolescents, as for anyone, there is a big difference between answering friends' questions or leading a class discussion about cancer, and suddenly, out of the blue and in a totally unrelated context, having a room full of people staring at you because you have cancer.

77

Finally, it's important to remember that teachers and their actions can be experienced as powerful forces in the lives of teenagers, despite frequent protests to the contrary.

PART FOUR

PLANNING FOR THE FUTURE

During adolescence, young people first begin to think seriously about what they want the rest of their lives to be like. Do they want a large family, small family, or no family at all? What careers best fit their particular interests?

High school students must at least decide whether or not to prepare to go on to college. Depending on their interests, some adolescents must do a lot more. Those wanting to be professional athletes, ballet dancers, or veterinarians, for example, have to make early commitments to these careers. As they well know, there are few chances in these professions for late developers. Most teenagers are not so sure, however, and are able to think of several attractive career possibilities.

Decisions about future careers affect plans for beginning a family, and, of course, a strong desire to start a family when young can in turn affect decisions about future employment. High school romances help adolescents refine their idea of what they want in a marriage partner, and, in fact, some teenagers actually find their future spouses in high school, either marrying them upon graduating or waiting a few years. Married or not, many young people begin their families as teenagers.

Getting cancer can throw a monkey wrench into

whatever plans the adolescent has made, although for most patients, the disruption is only temporary. Once recovered, they pick up their plans where they left off and continue with their lives. Their view of the future and how they want it to be remains relatively unchanged. These are the patients who have both a good prognosis and no lasting side effects from their treatment.

Other patients must change their plans. For some, treatment has left them physically unable to have the career they dreamed of or children of their own. For others, the possibility that they may not live long makes it hard to work for a future that they fear they will never see. Perhaps this is one of the most difficult tasks of all—to maintain the motivation to dream, plan, and work today for a tomorrow that might not come.

11

GETTING MARRIED AND RAISING A FAMILY

"I told my sister to get ready for me to spoil her kids a lot, 'cause that's what I'm going to do if I can't have any."

ANTHONY

"I've always wondered if I'd get married if I couldn't have kids, because that wouldn't be fair to the guy. I'm sure he'd want to make his own kids."

LAURA

In spite of the fact that teenage patients rarely ask about the effect of having cancer on their ability to have children, it is an area of great concern for them. Having learned that patients are usually reluctant to broach the topic, many physicians are careful to raise it themselves. "I always discuss it," said one oncologist, "and, believe me, as soon as I bring it up they're all ears!" In the vast majority of cases, doctors are able to reassure their patients that, once recovered, there is no reason why they can't have children. Oncologists are careful, however, to inform female patients about the dangers of getting pregnant while still on medication, because some of the drugs used to treat cancer can cause birth defects.

Most teenagers seem to assume that, at some time in their lives, they will settle down and raise a family. Although they may picture that day as very far in the future, they generally expect it to arrive at some point. Very few adolescents have decided that they definitely don't want to have children at all, whereas a number of them, boys as well as girls, are actively looking forward to having and caring for their own kids.

Dawn is really looking forward to having a baby. In her case, however, this event is only two months away. Shortly after getting off medication, Dawn met her first real boyfriend. When she discovered she was pregnant, both of them were very pleased. "Although Mark [her boyfriend] would rather it had been later, after I finished school," Dawn added. Mark plans to coach her through natural childbirth, and Dawn's family seems accepting of both her relationship with her boyfriend and her pregnancy.

Initially, however, Dawn was advised to have an abortion. The doctor who first told her she was pregnant also said that a pregnancy could cause her leukemia to recur. Frightened, Dawn called her oncologist, who assured her that was "nuts." Both Dawn and Mark would have been in favor of an abortion if her health had been endangered, but they are glad it wasn't necessary.

Did having cancer have anything to do with Dawn's getting pregnant as soon as she stopped her medication? In some instances, adolescents recently recovered from cancer need proof that they are normal and that they can still have children, and purposefully try to get pregnant. Sometimes, the first hint the oncologist has that the patient was worried about infertility is when he or she is confronted with a pregnant young woman. Such cases are very rare, however, and are becoming less frequent as doctors make sure that the topic of sterility and the patients' concerns about it are fully discussed. Although it's impossible to prove that these factors weren't influential in Dawn's situation, there's no reason to believe that she is any different from the many other fifteen-year-olds across the country who are also having babies.

Bernadette loves children and raising several of her own was something she just assumed she would do. Then, at fourteen, doctors discovered a tumor in her stomach and operated. Three days before leaving the hospital, her doctor told her that the tumor had "taken" one of her ovaries. Bernadette was extremely upset, but her doctor assured her that the remaining ovary would be enough to enable her to become pregnant. I told him, "Fine. You can do anything to me, but I want to have children!"

Two years later, when a "second look" operation indicated that it was necessary to remove her other ovary, Bernadette was devastated. "When I woke up [after the operation], I asked my mother if I had my ovary and she said, 'No.' I didn't believe it. I thought I was dreaming." It's not Bernadette's style, however, to waste time crying. Very pragmatically, she assessed her alternatives and realized that there were options she could live with. "I just told my doctor that I could put in for adoption when I turn eighteen." Since her uterus is intact, she might also consider implantation with an egg from her sister. "I was devastated, but I had other ways to go. If there hadn't been other alternatives, I think that would have been a real downfall, but there are." For Bernadette, raising children and having them to love are more important than actually bearing them herself, although that would be nice if possible.

"I want to have kids! Kids are awesome," Anthony said, his eyes glowing. "Some of the little kids you meet through friends are sharper than you think. I think a lot of little kids really have their acts together." It's apparent that Anthony both appreciates and enjoys children and looks forward to having them in his life. But, it's unlikely that the children Anthony raises will be his own. While making what seemed to be a grand tour of his body, cancer affected his reproductive organs. Treatment for this has probably left him sterile, although Anthony occasionally holds out faint hope that this isn't so. Basically, however, his interest in having children isn't in siring them but in nurturing them. Like Bernadette (and probably like many other fifteen-year-old boys, if they were asked), Anthony just adores kids. If he can't have his own, he'll adopt.

For Anthony and for Bernadette, facing the reality that they can't have their own children has been hard. But both have taken a look at what is important to them about raising a family and have adjusted their dreams accordingly. In a sense, for them, the problem has been solved.

For Laura, the whole issue is more complex. Her face lights up when she talks about children. "I could be really happy just being a mother. I don't even know if I can have kids, though, 'cause I've been on some medicine that can make you sterile. So that's another really sad thing."

Laura would like to find out one way or the other, but her mother discourages her. "There's a test you can have done. I'd really like to find out, but my mom just says, 'Laura, there's no need for you to know right now. You're not in a position to even want to have kids now.' "

True, but Laura feels that her fertility status will be important to her in deciding whether or not to get married. Almost twenty-one years old, she struggles with the question of whether it is fair to marry someone if you can't bear children. Some of her concern may also be self-protective. Over the years, she has learned that boyfriends often can't handle the problems associated with her illness, so she has become sensitized to the limitations cancer can place on relationships.

Even if she is able to have children, however, Laura isn't sure she should. At the moment, her prognosis is uncertain. Two recurrences have left her unsure as to how long she will live. Laura was especially affected by a scene in a recent movie in which a young mother dying of cancer and her little son said good-bye. Laura identified completely with the child and the thought of causing similar pain to her own children is unbearable. Thus, for a number of reasons, as much as she loves children, Laura doesn't know if she'll ever have a family.

12
CAREER PLANS

"I realized that even if I couldn't be an athlete anymore, I could still be almost anything I wanted."

KEVIN

"With school, sometimes it's a bit rough. You say, 'Why do I have to go through all this? In a couple of years, I'll probably die and it'll be a waste of time sitting here.'"

WINSTON

How does having cancer influence the career plans of adolescent patients? Do doctors and nurses become career role models that teenage patients want to emulate? Are there many jobs that a person who's had cancer can't do?

Considering the extensive exposure that cancer patients have to the medical world and the high regard patients generally have for the staff involved in their treatment, it's perhaps surprising that more teenagers aren't influenced by their experience and don't wish to enter the field of medicine. A few flirt with the idea, however. "When I first got sick," said Susan, "I thought about being a lab technician. But I really wanted to be a dental hygienist all along, so that's what I'm going to do." Derek toyed with the idea of becoming a doctor, but then decided it wasn't for him. "If you've been sick, you want to help other people . . . like be a social worker or a doctor. At first, I wanted to be a doctor, but I couldn't give those needles." Only Cheryl plans to be a nurse, but not because she had cancer. "I always wanted to be a nurse," she said, "even before I got sick."

Many teenage patients had already made some fairly firm career decisions before they got sick. While their plans may change over time, it probably won't be because they have had cancer. Gail especially likes working with word processors. She has wanted to be a secretary for a long time and plans to go to business school. Joel expects to go into engineering or perhaps computers—areas that interested him before he got sick. After thinking about being a doctor, Derek went back to his original plans. "I'm going to be a corporate lawyer somewhere in California, for a *big* corporation. Or something in computers." All three seem confident of their ability to achieve these plans and look forward to getting on with their futures.

For Bernadette, working for the future is what makes life worthwhile. She thrives on setting high goals for herself and then reaching them. Not surprisingly, she has some definite ideas about what she wants in terms of a career. "I want to be an accountant, a CPA," she said. "I'll work on passing my CPA exam until I'm eighty if I have to!"

For these young people, having cancer hasn't affected what they want to do with their lives or their ability to carry out their plans. Anthony, on the other hand, has had to modify his ideas about future work, but only slightly. When talking about what he hopes his life will be like when he's twenty-one, he says, only half joking, "I hope I'll be rich! I'll have my own car at least!" More seriously, he adds, "Possibly, I'll have finished a couple of years at a trade school . . . pipe fitting or something like that. I'd like to go back for accounting courses, something to start my own business."

Anthony thinks he might have tried to do construction work, but when treatment left him with no control over one foot, that idea had to be abandoned. Since he likes physical work that makes use of his mechanical abilities, pipe fitting will allow him to get the same satisfaction that a construction job would have provided. As a result, Anthony's not upset about having to adjust his plans.

Anthony hadn't considered going to college before he got sick, and he doesn't plan to go now. "I would have a tough time with college and that means waiting four more years before I start earning money. I want the bucks now!" he says, laughing. And Anthony doesn't see any reason why having had cancer should stop him.

Cancer stopped Kevin right in his tracks, however, ending all of his dreams. For as long as he can remember, he had wanted to become a professional athlete. His coach had told him that he was good enough to have a shot at it as well. Then Kevin's leg was amputated and his whole world fell apart. "I thought,

'What's the *point* of even being alive?' " For a while, he took out his anger on anyone around, including his parents and the hospital staff.

Slowly, though, Kevin began to see that there were other careers he could do that he might enjoy, even in sports. Since deciding to become a sports broadcaster, his life has picked up again. He feels interested in his new career choice and even has a television internship for the summer. It's been a long, hard haul, but Kevin thinks it's been worth it. Does he feel his plans for the future will work out? "Hey, I've been through a lot. I *deserve* to get what I want—and I think I will."

There are probably as many teenagers who don't know what they want to do in the future as there are those who have their career plans laid out. As Dawn puts it, "I think I've always wondered where I'll be in five years. Before this [cancer], I used to think, 'After I'm married and have kids, what will I be doing?' " Having cancer hasn't changed things. She still doesn't know. Nor do Earl, Amy, or Yvonne.

For other adolescents with cancer, the question isn't *what* to do but *why* to do it. Winston's very clear about his plans for the future. "I'd like to finish my education and go into something in communications . . . I wanted to be a journalist, but I hate reading and writing. I could tell the story but not write it, so I went into radio." Although only nineteen, he's already had an off-air job with a major FM station.

The trouble is that Winston doesn't have much reason to think he'll live to do the things he's planned. Reminders such as the constant pain he suffers and the bleak survival statistics for his type of cancer make it difficult for him to ignore the possibility that he may die. Not knowing whether his efforts will pay off saps his motivation to work hard in school. On the other hand, Winston doesn't want to quit planning and working for his future because, who knows? He might live. Whenever he's on the verge of just taking it easy, he tells himself, "You should do this [school] because you don't know what the future holds."

Laura experiences the same conflict. "Some people say to me, 'Laura, why do you want to go to college if you're going to die?' Well, what do you want me to do? Waste away my life and then I'll have nothing accomplished and when I die, it'll be like, 'Well, what did she do with her life? Oh, she goofed it all away.' So, I have to do things, to plan for a future, if I'm going to have one."

Does she believe she'll have a future? "I don't know. Sometimes I do, sometimes I don't. It's hard to always be on a positive note." Most of the time she manages to stay hopeful. "I'd like to work for a large corporation doing public relations work and volunteer coordinating events for the Leukemia Society or the Cancer Society. I thought I wanted to do that [cancer work] full time, but you get really stagnant in that and the salary isn't great. But I *do* think I'm going to do it almost all the time, and then. . . ."

PART FIVE

COMING TO TERMS

In many respects, having cancer is a very personal experience. It affects every aspect of patients' lives, from their relationships with friends to their relationships with their own bodies. Cancer forces teenagers to face sometimes overwhelming fears of isolation, pain, and death, at a period in life when, for most people, these issues couldn't be more remote. The experience also touches adolescent patients at a particularly important time in the development of their own values and sense of self and, to varying degrees, helps shape them as individuals.

In spite of their very different personalities and backgrounds, the young people who helped in the writing of this book were very similar in one respect. They all showed a remarkable willingness to share their lives, often in very intimate terms, so that we might better understand what having cancer is really like.

13
WHAT IF I DIE?

"I think I never accepted the fact, when they said, 'If you don't do this, you're going to die.' I just didn't believe that."

DEREK

"It's hard when a friend dies and you go and you look at them at a wake and some of them had the same disease you have—that makes it a little real for a second, but not forever."

LAURA

Although younger cancer patients fear death primarily in terms of separation from their parents, adolescent patients are old enough to understand, and fear, death itself. At precisely the time when they are beginning to explore the many exciting possibilities their futures may hold, teenagers with cancer are slapped in the face with the prospect of having no future at all. Because of the nature of cancer, all patients old enough to have a concept of death struggle, at one point or another, with the idea that their disease may kill them.

How they handle this frightening possibility varies as much as the individuals themselves.

Confrontation with the possibility of dying begins the moment patients are told their diagnoses. For many, the very word cancer is synonymous with death. Even when patients themselves don't immediately recognize the dire implications of their illness, the panic and distress of their parents or others quickly cue them in to the knowledge that something devastating has occurred. Anthony's father felt that he should be the one to tell his son that he had cancer. He got three words out and burst into tears. Nothing could have made it clearer to Anthony that he was in real trouble.

Even after learning that they have cancer, patients don't always relate this to the fact that they may die. They are soon made aware of the connection, however. Although she knew she had a bone tumor that would require surgery, Amy was shocked when, at her initial meeting with the oncology team, the possibility of her death was raised. "They were talking about how they hoped that this would just be two years of my life that I'd want to forget, and if I survived . . . and I said, 'SURVIVE? What do you mean, *survive?*' My father had been saying, 'It's OK, everything will be fine,' and the hospital even said, 'Don't get upset until we have the results,' and now they were saying, 'if you survive.' I walked out!"

How patients handle this initial realization that they might die depends to a great extent on their prognosis. When physicians can honestly tell them that their chances of survival are good, or very good, patients' fears of dying subside dramatically. Susan's first thought when she heard she had cancer was, "I wonder how much longer I have to live." When told that her type of cancer was curable in 90 percent of the cases, both she and her parents began to relax a little.

It's only been a few months since Gail was diagnosed as having cancer. When asked if she ever worried that she might die, she answered, "In the beginning," but then started to cry softly. After a few moments, she added, "But after listening to all the doctors and nurses telling me everything was going to be all right, it was fine." Gail's parents have tried to help allay her fears, but they're still grappling with some of their own. "My parents reassured me that I would be fine if I go through with treatment."

A diagnosis of cancer is a tremendous shock to the entire family, shattering everyone's sense of security. Patients, parents, and siblings all need time to reestablish their equilibrium and to understand and accept the implications of the disease. Those teenagers with cancer that can be successfully treated incorporate their doctors' encouraging statistics and assurances into their own outlook, push their fears into the background, and assume they will survive. This approach is appropriate, since they are likely to live, and it enables them to get the most out of their lives.

Patients' beliefs that they will be all right and that they won't die can be shaken by other events. Obviously, patients whose disease recurs are forced to face the fact that they aren't getting better. But recurrences in other patients, particularly if they are fatal and occur in those who appeared to have recovered, remind all patients that death can strike even those who seem to be improving. Cheryl had become very close to Sara and was extremely upset by her friend's death. "I was really sad, really unhappy, because she had gotten *well* so I thought it was going to be all right."

Amy wants to believe what she's been told by the medical staff, who say encouraging things about her prognosis. But she's not blind. The three people she's known with her diagnosis have all died, including a girl who had been disease-free for eight years. Although these deaths may be atypical, they're what Amy sees and she's having difficulty reconciling these events with her own supposedly good chances of survival.

On the other hand, examples of people who have had cancer and are doing well can help adolescent patients believe that they can also recover. It means something to Earl to see that Edward Kennedy's son, who also had osteogenic sarcoma and an amputation, is still surviving and living a normal life. Closer to home, his grandmother, who has had cancer twice, tells him, "See, I haven't given up and I've had it twice. Don't give up, no matter what!"

A few patients completely deny the life-threatening implications of their illness. At one point or another, these defenses tend to break down. "It runs in my family to be a rock, a stone, to take care of others," Joel said. Most of his friends see him as courageous, able to face cancer without fear. But when one girl told him, "It's not that you're so brave, it's just that you don't deal with it," Joel broke down and cried. "It was the first time I really thought about all of it, about the possibility of dying," he said.

When patients' chances of surviving are not great, however, they must realistically come to terms with the possibility that they could die, while at the same time not give up the life and future they may have. Laura tries not to think about it and to go about her life as if she'll be here forever. But, sometimes when she least expects it, the possibility of dying pops into her mind. "My birthday's next week and I know my dad will say, 'What do you want?' and I thought of telling him that I wanted a ski sweater. And real quick, it went through my mind, 'What if I die before I get to use the ski sweater? Maybe I should get something that I want to use this summer.' And then I thought, 'Laura, don't think like that!' "

Winston knows he's battling lousy odds. "When the doctors would tell me the statistics, I just said, 'Wow!' They said that one out of ten survives. They don't live past three years . . . So on their thinking about it, I've gone one year and I have two more to go. Then after the two years, if I'm here, it'll be like I beat the thing." In the meantime, he plans his funeral, just in case. "I told her [his mother] how I'd like it to be, if I died. I told her where I want to be buried, who I want there, how I want it done. I want people to walk away going, 'Boy, that was a good funeral! That was like a Broadway performance!' "

Winston doesn't want his friends to make a big deal

about his illness. "They're taking it OK. They know and it's like, I don't talk about it and they don't talk about it." When his friends express anxiety that he might die, Winston deflects their fears by joking. "If I didn't come to school for a couple of weeks, people would come up to me and say, 'I'm glad you came to school 'cause I thought you died.' They'd be saying, 'Please, let him come to school.' I'd say, 'No, I'm still here. If I die you'll be the first to know . . . I'll send the invitations out.'"

Although Laura lives with the awareness that she may die, other family members are constantly preoccupied with the possibility, placing her under a lot of stress. "My mom's always so worried that I'm going to die. And my sister, Joanne, she daydreams a lot and in her daydreams, she always visualizes whether it's before or after I've died." Dealing with their fears and the effect she feels her death would have on them has been very hard for Laura. "I really don't think I could ever, ever give up completely, because I know my mother and Joanne couldn't handle it. That's one of the biggest pressures that there is. Whenever I want to give up, I know that Joanne and my mom are still going to be here. My mother would have to clean out my room, and Joanne wouldn't be able to get along. That's a lot of pressure."

Perhaps because she was sick for so long and in the hospital so frequently, Laura has seen many cancer patients die. Yet, even for her, death—her own death—remains unreal. Maybe this is what makes it tolerable to live in such close proximity with the possibility of dying. "Well, it's *never real*. Even to me now. I mean, how can you visualize yourself dying? It's never really real. I was talking to a fifteen-year-old, and he said, 'It doesn't seem real.' And I said, 'It never will, kid!' "

14

LOOKING AT MYSELF

"It's made me a better, more compassionate person."

KEVIN

"Well, it brought my family closer together. We talked a lot more. Before, I was never open about my feelings with my family."

GAIL

Having cancer means dealing with a life-threatening illness for a couple of years, perhaps longer. It means facing pain and loneliness, feeling ugly, and, sometimes, losing a limb. It may mean seeing friends die. It always means worrying, at least some of the time, about dying yourself. How does this experience—cancer—affect teenagers? Not just their lives, but them as human beings. Are they different now from what they would have been if they'd never had cancer?

While having cancer is unquestionably a significant life event, adolescents vary greatly in how their personalities and outlooks are affected by the experience. Clearly, each individual's belief system and style of coping have a great deal to do with how the experience of cancer will be understood and incorporated into the person's sense of self.

Dawn feels that cancer caused certain aspects of her to change dramatically, but, in accordance with her religion, she attributes these changes to the fact that during treatment she underwent a transfusion with a stranger's blood. "I used to run track, but now I can't run anymore. I don't know what happened. It's probably the blood they gave me. It's from somebody else. It changed my personality." Gradually, her own new blood cells have replaced the transfused blood and she feels that she's "going back to my old self again."

Bernadette doesn't think that having had cancer has changed her, as a person, at all. A girl whose style is action-oriented rather than introspective, Bernadette's awareness of people, including herself, is based more on what they do and what they make of themselves than on an abstract idea of who they are. Highly competitive, she enjoys overcoming obstacles. In her eyes, cancer was just another one of these challenges. "It [cancer] was just another injury I had during my life. If you don't have trouble establishing yourself in life, then it comes too easy. You have to work for what you're worth."

Bernadette thought of the whole experience of having cancer as an external contest that could be won or lost but not as an event likely to shape her personality. Thus, while she is pleased at having won (an outcome she never doubted), she doesn't feel changed by the experience. She does consider the experience to have had some important positive consequences for her, though. "It was a time that I wouldn't want to forget, that I can't forget, because it's an experience I've learned a lot from and I feel I can help other people."

Most teenagers feel their bout with cancer has had a more long-term, personal effect on them, influencing their personalities, their outlook on life, and/or their relationships with other people. Almost always, they see these changes as positive. "Before I got sick," said Amy, "I was kind of snobby to people. Being sick made me appreciate what is important in life. I think I'm more considerate of other people. Yeah, more caring and more considerate."

Derek found, like Gail, that having cancer brought him closer to his family, while Joel felt that having cancer affected the way he looked at life. "I have a much better perspective on problems, on life in general now. I'm more aware of the good things in life." Being able to cope with her illness enhanced Susan's sense of her own abilities. "It's made me a stronger person," she said. "I'm able to handle more things now."

Laura feels these same effects but at a deeper level. For her, cancer is not an experience that she is passing through but something that has molded her as a person. "I think it's *made* me what I am. I think it does everybody." Since Laura has had cancer for so long, it's perhaps not surprising that she feels its influence in her personality more intensely. After all, it's been a bigger part of her life. Years of struggling with a serious disease have made her a lot stronger and a lot more understanding toward other people's handicaps too. "Like someone in a wheelchair—I don't feel sorry for them anymore 'cause they're still happy even if they have a problem. I've learned to make the most of things."

In case these young people begin to sound unbelievably optimistic, it's important to remember that, although they can cite positive things that have come out of their cancer experience, all would have preferred to forgo the whole thing. As Laura points out, they just have learned to find the good things in a basically miserable experience. And, for all of them, there have been times when it was very difficult indeed to dig up anything that could be considered good. That is how Winston is feeling now. In constant pain, he can see absolutely nothing positive in having cancer except, as he says wryly, "Maybe I'll get a phone call from Michael Jackson."

15
LAST THOUGHTS

If you ask teenage cancer patients what they would like others to know most of all about the experience of having cancer and about people who have cancer, certain themes come up over and over again. Although some of these issues have been touched on in one form or another in earlier chapters, this chapter is intended to emphasize these themes in the way the adolescents who discussed them intended.

TO OTHER CANCER PATIENTS

> *"Live your life to the fullest, take one day at a time, don't think people should treat you differently—act like yourself."*
>
> KEVIN

> *"Think positive, that you will make it. Take your medicine. Don't let the medicine overwhelm you. It's your body, you control your body, you can overrun it. Just think positive and don't ever give up. Just keep saying you're going to make it."*
>
> CHERYL

"It's not forever. It will get better. You should have a positive attitude."

SUSAN

"Do the best you can to be strong, more emotionally but physically too. Take into consideration that no matter how bad it gets, sooner or later it's got to stop. If you let it hurt real bad for a certain period of time, before long it can't be bad at all."

ANTHONY

"Don't worry about it that much. Go on living."

EARL

"A bad attitude can make you feel worse. Try to get your mind off it and get well. Moping around will make you sicker."

BERNADETTE

"It's nothing you can't overcome. Take the attitude that nothing has really happened. You'll notice that there are some nights you can't sleep because you'll think, 'Gosh, each day now is really very special. You have to live that day to the fullest.' You'll have this [leukemia] for a long time, but you won't feel it every day. You have pain one day, the next day you'll be fine. Don't pay it any mind."

WINSTON

109

To Other People

"FRIENDSHIP MAKES THE DIFFER-
ENCE! *It makes you fight harder.*"

KEVIN

"*We're not different. We're the same people [that we were before we got sick].*"

GAIL

"*I certainly wish people were a little less
afraid. The reality of cancer is not nearly as
frightening as the fantasy.*"

BETH

"*Three things: (1) Other kids were afraid to
ask about my wig, or cancer, or anything.
But I could see their eyes constantly going
up to my wig. This bothered me more than
if they did ask questions. It creates a barrier
not to ask. (2) Let the person with cancer
keep a normal life. If they need help, they'll
ask for it. (3) The most important thing is
your friends!*"

JOEL

"*Just treat them [people who have cancer]
the same. If you didn't treat them well in
the first place, just treat them a little better
than you did before.*"

DEREK

"*People need to learn that cancer doesn't
mean dying.*"

LAURA

110

GLOSSARY

Bone marrow The spongy, jelly-like material that fills the cavities of bone.

Cancer A general term for about one hundred diseases characterized by the uncontrolled growth and spread of abnormal cells.

Chemotherapy The treatment of cancer using cell-killing drugs.

Hematologist A person specializing in the study of blood diseases.

Intravenous (IV) The administration of a drug or fluid directly into a vein.

Leukemia The term for a variety of cancers that arise in blood and bone marrow cells.

Lymphoma Cancers that affect white blood cells of the immune system. Lymphomas are usually classified as Hodgkin's disease or non-Hodgkin's lymphomas.

Malignant Cancerous.

Oncologist A physician specializing in the treatment of cancer.

Oncology The study of cancer.

Osteogenic sarcoma The most common bone cancer in children, arising at the ends of bones, particularly the large bones of the leg and upper arm.

Prosthesis An artificial replacement for a missing part of the body. In the case of adolescent cancer patients, usually an artificial leg.

Radiation The treatment of disease with X-ray, radium, or other radioactive materials.

Spinal tap Insertion of a needle into the spinal canal to draw out fluid for diagnosis or to administer drugs.

Tumor An abnormal growth. Tumors can be either benign (noncancerous) or malignant (cancerous). When used in this book, the term refers to a cancerous growth unless otherwise specified.

SUGGESTED FURTHER READING

Fox, Ray Errol. *Angela Ambrosia.* New York: Alfred A. Knopf, 1979.

Harris, Gail Kay. *Cancer.* New York: Franklin Watts, 1980.

Pendleton, Edith. *Too Old to Cry, Too Young to Die.* Nashville: Thomas Nelson. 1980.

The following books can be obtained free of charge by writing:

The National Cancer Institute
Building 31, Room 10A18
Bethesda, MD 20205

Help Yourself—Tips for Teenagers with Cancer
Taking Time—Support for People with Cancer and the People Who Care About Them
What You Need to Know About Cancer
What You Need to Know About Leukemia
Medicine for the Layman—Cancer Treatment

INDEX

ABOUT THE AUTHORS

KAREN GRAVELLE was born in Alexandria, Virginia. She received an MSW from Catholic University and a Ph.D. in biopsychology from the City University of New York. Dr. Gravelle has written several books for children and is the co-author of *Deciphering the Senses*, a book on sensory systems for the general public. She is currently the senior science editor at Fox Chase Cancer Center in Philadelphia.

BERTRAM A. JOHN is a psychologist specializing in cognitive/social development. He was born in the eastern Caribbean island of St. Vincent and earned his Ph.D. at Rutgers University. Dr. John was previously professor of psychology at Montclair State College and coordinator of Afro-American studies there. Currently, he is at St. Mary's Hospital of Brooklyn, where he is responsible for staff training.